Health Facilitation & Health

MEETING THE HEALTH
PEOPLE WITH LEARNING
DISABILITIES in one London area.

CW00746188

Musthafar Giwa Oladosu B.sc RNMH, RN(MH), M.A

A Dissertation submitted in partial fulfillment of the requirements for the award of M.A
(Health and Social Care Management) of the
London Metropolitan University, London
HSPP05N
Policy Implementation Evaluation Project

Submitted on 8th of September 2006

"A very good dissertation. A good range of reading, clearly structured answer, accurately referenced. A good analysis of the rationale for the policy chosen, including level and type of need and demand, locally. Good engagement with service needs, and how to achieve them, you have a sound grasp of both policy and practice which is fluently articulated. Some further engagement and analysis of the research cited would lead to even higher marks. Well done." Lecturer & Marker

NB: This is a self publication for work submitted as a dissertation. The writer has added some new materials to the original work under *post script*. Though, considerable effort has been made to ensure that this work is completely flawless with regards to grammar and accuracy of evidence used, the extent to which this has been achieved is for reader to judge. Prior apology is given for any flaw.

To Lara, Morin, Folabi and Folarin

Acknowledgement

I give special thanks and gratitude to my dissertation supervisor – Ms Carina Browne. I acknowledge her support, advice and guidance throughout this work. Her objective criticisms were always illuminative whenever my own search light was too weak to help me see beyond my nose. I wish her all the best for the future as she retires.

I also thank my employers for giving me the opportunity and funding to study for this M.A in Health and Social Care Management. And to my Manager whose understanding helped me to combine this academic work with my job and professional responsibilities. Unfortunately, due to ethical and confidential considerations their names cannot be mentioned in this acknowledgement.

I am also indebted to my colleagues at neighbouring Community Learning Disabilities Teams (CLDT) in London who hosted me, gave me their time and shared with me their practice experience and views on how their teams were implementing *Valuing People* health agenda for people with learning disabilities. I salute their passion and commitment to working with people with learning disabilities to live healthier lives and receive same quality healthcare as everybody else. Above all, I give gratitude to God. I acknowledge His past, present and future blessings.

Table of Contents

Abstract

In 2001, the Government came up with *Valuing People: A Strategy for Learning Disability in the 21ˢᵗ Century*. This was the first White paper in this area for thirty years and it was part of the New Labour government inclusion agenda and modernisation of health and social services in England.

In the White Paper the Government acknowledged that people with learning disabilities have poorer health and that they receive poorer services from the health services. Health Facilitation and Health Action Planning were the two main strategies which government proposed to address this apparent health inequality which this population experience. Each local Specialist Learning Disabilities team is expected to implement these strategies.

In this dissertation the writer examines how a local learning disabilities team implemented Health Facilitation and Health Action Planning. The writer compares the local implementation with implementation in some other areas of London and nationally and found that there is wide divergence in how strategies to improve the health needs of people with learning disabilities are been implemented across the country.

Introduction

This dissertation examines the health needs of people with learning disabilities and how a local Community Learning Disabilities Team (CLDT) in London worked to meet the health needs of this population. The dissertation is anchored on the established research findings that people with learning disabilities experience more health inequalities compared to the general population. The Government White Paper *Valuing People: A new strategy for learning disabilities in the 21st century* (Department of Health 2001), henceforth referred to simply as *Valuing people*, is a government attempt to deal comprehensively with socio-economic and health barriers this population faces. It is a whole life Social inclusion agenda in which positive health is the foundation (Greig 2003).

There will be an analysis and discussions of how *Valuing People* was implemented locally and nationally with particular reference to Health Facilitation and Health Action planning which are the two main strategies that the White Paper proposed under its chapter on health titled: Improving Health for People with Learning disabilities.

Chapter one is the result of extensive, literature search and review on the health needs of people with learning disabilities and the health inequalities they experience. The writer aims to appreciate and draw from existing knowledge and at the same time demonstrate own understanding of the core issues in this dissertation.

In chapter two the writer explains and discusses research methodology used in this dissertation. The chapter also lays out the aims of this research work and the methods that the writer used to achieve stated aims of the study.

In chapter three the writer takes an historical perspective on the trends in care provision for people with learning disabilities in Britain. This chapter provides background to the new thinking in the service provision for this client group.

Chapter four reviews the *Valuing People* proposed health strategies – Health Facilitation and Health Action Planning. Here these twin strategies are defined, explained and discussed.

Chapter five deals with how Health Facilitation and Health Action Planning are being implemented in one area of London. In this chapter, the writer identifies local organisational and management issues in relation to the implementation of the strategies in the area of study. The writer also tried to compare implementation of these strategies in the area of study with other areas of London.

In the conclusion, the writer sums up the key research findings in this dissertation. The dissertation ends with some recommendations to improve the implementation of Health Facilitation and Health Action Planning in the local areas. Some of these recommendations may also be relevant to other similar areas in the country.

Chapter One
Health Needs of People with Learning Disabilities: A Theoretical perspective and Review of literature

Clarifying terminologies: *Learning disability*
In the United Kingdom the term learning disabilities was adopted as it was felt that it conveys less negative image than other previous terms. It was an attempt to accurately describe difficulties experienced by the people who have this condition (Mackean et all 1999). It is a terminology that was coined in the mid 80s to refer to condition which used to be referred to as *idiocy, imbecility, mental sub normality, mental handicap* and *mental deficiency* (Kelly 2000). Other terms which are used in some literature are *developmental disability, intellectual impairment, cognitive disability, learning difficulties and mental retardation.* This plethora of terminologies and lack of agreement on one has brought about confusion especially when group of practitioners in the field meet with colleagues from the other part of the world (Kelly 2000). For instance, learning disabilities appeared to be used only in the United Kingdom and to some extent in the Republic of Ireland. Even then some writers in these countries prefer to use *intellectual* or *cognitive disability.* While in the United States and the United Nations, mental retardation is still the official terminology. The situation makes literature search more cumbersome and laborious. In this work the author has adopted learning disability reflecting the official term used by the British government and the Department of Health and the Social Services Department.

Despite lack of unity in terminology, there appears to be universal agreement among writers on what this condition is regardless of the terminology used to refer to it. World Health Organisation (1993 cited in Kelly 2000) defines is it as a condition of arrested or incomplete development of the mind, which starts at early developmental period leading to significant impairment in skills. It also affects overall intelligence i.e. cognitive, language, motor and social abilities. Similarly, the Department of Health (2001) defined learning disabilities as presence of:

Significantly reduced ability to understand new or complex information, to learn new skills (impaired intelligence), with a reduced ability to cope independently (impaired social functioning, which started before adulthood, with a lasting effect on development.

Learning disabilities is the most common form of disability in the United Kingdom and the least understood (See Mencap web site http://www.mencap.org.uk/html/about_learning_disability) The Department of Health (2001) estimated that there are about 210,000 people with severe and profound learning disabilities out of which 65,000 children and young people, 120,000 adults of working age and 25,000 older people. However, people with mild to moderate learning disabilities are estimated to be about 1.2 million in England alone. The Department of Health reported that prevalence of severe and profound learning disabilities is distributed fairly and uniformly across England and socio-economic groups, while in the case of mild to moderate learning disability there is a link to poverty and that rate are higher in the deprived areas.

Health

Health does not let itself to easy or universally acceptable definition. Saunders (2003) argued that health is so difficult to define in a way that reflects individual views, perceptions and circumstances. The problem of establishing a common definition of health has made the concept to assume what Saunders (2003 p. 24) described as "momentous importance and complete insignificance" The reason for this paradox is not difficult to figure out. Health has assumed eminence in so far as it has attracted world wide attention from experts, practitioners, governments and organisations at all levels, they look at multidimensional nature of health in relation to policy and strategy formulation aimed at shaping citizens' health. On the other hand however, it can be argued that what health really means is irrelevant and insignificant as health is simply what individual perceives it to mean for him/her. The important thing to note is that everybody has a view on what health means.

However, it would be useful for the purpose of service design, investment and delivery, in terms of care planning and interventions to gain a compromise definition which at least most people would feel comfortable with.

Health is often seen from two dominant perspectives – medical and social models of health. A medical model which is also sometimes referred to in literature as bio-medical model, sees health as the absence of disease (Mackean 1999), a state of recognisable pathology, a deviation from normal biological functioning which can be identified and treated . The human body is likened to a machine which has repairable and replicable parts (Bowling 2002).This explains why physicians see their role from ancient Greek as that of treating disease to restore health and by correcting imperfections caused by the accidents of birth or life (Dubos 1960 cited in Towsend & Davidson 1982). Towsend & Davidson (1982) earlier observed that health as a word is derived from an English word which means 'whole' and that it is object of healing process which in turn leads to being whole and restoring health. However, focus on disease can lead to people with disabilities and chronic illnesses being labelled as sick or diseased when they may in fact be healthy. Medical perspective has also been criticised as minimalist and simplistic (Mackean et al 1999).

The social model of health on the other hand locates the individual within an environment and adopts a multi-causal perspective to determinants of health and illness. The model steps out of the body to stress the roles of politics, economic, social psychology, culture, environment as well as biological factors. For instance poor housing, poverty, prejudice and discrimination are known factors in poor health (Acheson 2000) and many people with disabilities experience these in greater degree. The social model takes the subjective experience of individual living into account. In fact, pioneers of social models are largely individuals with disabilities who were able to draw from their personal experiences (Barnes 1998)

In 1946 the World Health Organisation (WHO 1946 cited in Saunders 2001) provided, perhaps, the most widely cited definition which described health as "a state of complete physical, mental and social well-being, and not merely the absence of disease or infirmity". WHO went on to argue that enjoyment of highest quality of health is a fundamental right of every human being regardless of race, religion, political beliefs, economic or social status. This definition 50 years on is still attracting comments and criticisms. Some argued that the definition is utopian and idealistic (Saunders 2001 & Bowling 2002) hence unachievable. Yet, this definition remains the closest to a universally acceptable definition of health there is. The reason for this may be due in part to the fact that the definition attempted to combine both medical and social model of health and illness.

Good health can be seen as , absence of bodily pains, discomfort and distress even beyond what can be treated or cured through manipulation of bodily organs. This is why Towsend & Davidson (1982) argued that positive expression of vigour and wellbeing which enable one to engage with ones environment or community is good health. It then follows that poor health is interruption or inability to gain such vigour to the extent that one is unable to take full advantage of ones environment. This is consistent with the DoH (2004 pp. 1) assertion that "good health and well being is fundamental to us all, enabling us to live active, fulfilled lives". The issue of what health means to people with learning disabilities themselves has not attracted much research attention.

Health inequalities amongst people with learning disabilities

Achieving a universal definition of health is problematic, recognition that good health is not evenly shared (Woodward & Kawachi 2000) among and across all sections of the society appeared to be less controversial. Murray (1999) observed that social group or population differ, based on biological, social, economic and geographical characteristics. Whilst Peters (2006) argued that inequalities in health and access to uptake of health services remained an ongoing problem. Peters argued that the gap between the best and the least has increased in the last two decades. This is against the backdrop of social and medical advancements in our society. Health Development Agency (2004 pp. 2) described a paradox in Britain where comparatively speaking, collectively the country is healthier "than it has ever being in history" when one considers the fact that life expectancy has improved, prevalence of killer diseases have decreased as a result of advances in preventive approaches to public health and treatments. Yet, the problem of health inequality has refused to go away. Graham & Kelly (2004) concluded that while the health of the population on the whole may be improving that of less well off either improves more slowly than the rest of the population or even gets worse.

Acheson (2000) while making similar claim regarding the paradox of health inequalities in Britain stressed that the problem is pervasive in all stages of life from pregnancy to old age.

Health inequality is therefore a term used to describe the fact that health varies between individuals. It is a systematic difference in health between groups occupying unequal social economic position in society (Graham 2004). Health inequality suggests that some people due to factors such as poverty, race, and other social economic and or disabilities which are often beyond these people's control, carry heavier burden of ill health than other people and prevent them from accessing quality of health care possible or available to other people in the same society. This is why health inequality leads to moral judgment and question of fairness which are consistent with the concept of equity.

Lin et al (2004) defined inequity as disadvantages due to geographical area, age, cultural and social background, and kind of disability or illness. Lin et al (2004) argued that search for health equity should concern fairness in terms of arrangement for funding, purchasing and delivery of health care including the spread, ease of access to services as well as appropriateness of such services. This argument is particularly relevant to people with learning disabilities whose needs and presentations are often outside what the mainstream health care providers are accustomed to.

There is recognition that people with learning disabilities are disadvantaged group of people. If one adopts Whitehead (2000) argument that health inequalities are differential health experiences that are unnecessary and avoidable to the extent that they are unjust and unfair, it then becomes apparent that what many people with learning disabilities experience, is more consistent with health inequity than just health inequalities. Disability Right Commission (2006) conducted a formal investigation into health experience of people with mental health problems and people with learning disabilities in Britain. In its interim report titled "Equal Treatment: Closing the gap" the Commission acknowledged that there is a significant research evidence showing that these group of people are more likely to die young and to live with physical ill health than other citizens. The Commission found that often the physical health problems in this population are potentially preventable. Yet, these health problems tend to shorten lives and reduce life chances in this population.

Kavachi et al 2002 takes a different perspective and argues that health inequality is both inevitable and necessary. This line of argument maintains that individual responsibilities and choices play significant roles in the nature of health disadvantages they face, rather than deliberate systematic inequalities rooted in the system or society as a whole. While there may be some merit in this argument with reference to the general population, such argument, strictly speaking, misses the point about the impact of physical, mental and or cognitive disabilities on individuals, as well as societal responses and prejudice on the health experience of people with learning disabilities. Whitehead (2002) however argues that as a result of lack of resources, poorer social groups' living circumstances leave them with little or no safeguard but to experience higher ill health. It was further argued that sense of injustice is heightened in such cases as problems such as housing problem, poor financial status, communication problems and prejudice tend to cluster together and reinforce each other leaving the individual with little or no control. In this respect, Acheson (2000) argued that because health inequalities is largely due to factors outside individual responsibilities, the agent usually held responsible for identifying and rectifying the problem is the state. Literature revealed (Alborz et al 2003) that despite advances and progress that have been made in almost all areas of care of people with learning disabilities they continue to face wide range of barriers when accessing health services.

Research (Mackean 1999, Hortwitz et al 2000 Department of Health 2002, Alborz 2005, Disability Right Commission 2006, Health Care Commission 2006) has shown that people with learning disabilities are more prone to experiencing a wide range of physical and mental health problems than the general population and that they utilise health services less than the general population (Department of Health 1995). Evidence from the United States also confirmed that health needs of people with learning disabilities tend to be complex and on-going. They are likely to receive inappropriate and inadequate treatment or be denied health care altogether (US Public Health Service 2002).

Evidence from the literature (Holins et al 1998) indicates that respiratory disease is the primary health problem for people with learning disabilities accounting for around 50% of deaths compared to 15% in the general population. And over 50% of people with learning disabilities who have Downs Syndrome are affected by congenital heart problems, hypothyroidism and early onset dementia (Howel 1986 cited in Alborz, Brookes & Alberman 1996). Research carried out by Halton et al (2004) indicated that this group of people die at a younger age than the general population, they have 58% chances of dying by the age of 50. Incidence of cancer in people with learning disabilities is reported to be on the increase, while they have 48% - 58.5% of developing gastrointestinal cancer compared to 25% in the general population. Halton (2004) research further showed that people with learning disabilities only have 17% chances of receiving cervical smear test compared to 77% chances of general population. 22% have epilepsy compared to 0.4 – 1% in the general population. Other common health problems found in this population are poorer health hygiene, higher incidence of obesity, poorer dietary intake, higher incidence of sensory impairment and mental health problems. Despite this reported higher prevalence of many medical conditions in this population, the Health Care Commission (2006) pointed out that people with learning disabilities tend to be excluded from the general screening services and are not routinely identified in the information systems that monitor public health.

Many reasons have been given to explain the poorer health status of people with learning disabilities and why they continue to encounter barriers and difficulties when accessing required health services. Though, generally speaking, the factors at play in the health experience of people with learning disabilities are similar to those of the general population. The nature and level of individual disabilities in terms of associated biological predisposition which are associated with some types of learning disabilities, level of cognitive and adaptive skills and abilities including communication difficulties tend to compound these factors in this population. The United States Public Health Service (2001) claimed that because of complexity of health needs and the nature of individual learning disabilities many health providers avoid them in the State.

Shaughnessy & Cruse (2001) classified barriers which people with learning disabilities face into two categories: professional barriers and client barriers.

Professional barriers: It is argued that health care professionals are neither familiar with people with learning disabilities as a population, nor with their health needs. The implication is that mainstream health care professionals especially in primary health care and acute health services lack the knowledge and skills to meet identified needs (Kerr et al 1996, Bond et al 1997). Even in some cases health needs go unidentified leading to serious consequences including death (Kerr 1998). Attitude of health professionals towards people with learning disabilities has also been blamed. Many health care professionals see people with learning disabilities as a "special" group requiring specialist services (Bond et al 1997). The danger in this attitude is that people with learning disabilities are prone to falling between two types of health care systems without receiving either. Mackean (1999) stressed that primary care services are the 'linchpin' and the first point of health service provision as it comprised General Medical Practitioners (GPs), District Nurses, Health Visitors, and Practice Nurses among others and it is therefore best suited to tackle multiple health needs of this population. Yet, Kerr (1996 cited in Mackean et al 1999) argued that there is evidence that while the GPs accept that they should meet the primary health needs of people with learning disabilities, they do not accept that they should engage in health promotion work such as offering regular health checks for this client group. Other problems are poor communication skill of GPs in relation to people with learning disabilities. GPs' difficulties to provide suitable consultation appointment times or home visits and crowded waiting rooms are recognised by the Department of Health (1999). It needs to be stressed that people with learning disabilities experience similar and perhaps more complex barriers when accessing acute secondary health care services including mental health services. Of particular importance is the physical layout of many hospitals which may be inaccessible for people with additional physical disabilities or those with significant behaviour difficulties. Complex process of consultation and treatment are not helped by information systems that are often difficult for people with learning disabilities to understand (NHS Service Delivery Organisation 2004)

At the individual level is the nature and the impact of cognitive deficit arising from the presence of learning disabilities itself. Many people with learning disabilities have significant communication and language difficulties, hence they often lack the ability to articulate and communicate symptoms they experience. Many are unable to actively participate and influence their treatment options. Cognitive impairment may also make it difficult for a learning disabled adult to pick up vital ill health clues that are going on in his or her body and act on this by seeking professional help or make necessary adjustment to lifestyle and behaviour promptly. It has also been argued that preventive health promotion work such as cervical screening and weight management and healthy eating for instance may be problematic for many people with learning disabilities as they may find it difficult to appreciate these interventions as a ways of preventing or detecting bigger problem that might arise. Mackean (1999) observed that this may explain in part why people with learning disabilities are often excluded from such screening which the general population benefits from.

Inevitably, many people with learning disabilities rely on other people such as paid and unpaid carers who help them to navigate complex network of health care system. Alborz et al (2005) in their study, claimed that though the role of carers is to recognise symptoms or indicators of abnormal health, to secure access to health care facilities, to interpret and communicate with care providers and to support and encourage treatment compliance, they often themselves lack the knowledge and skills that are necessary to play this role effectively. It has been pointed out that carers from ethnic minority groups whose first language is not English face even tougher challenges in advocating effectively for their learning disabled member of their family (Department of Health 2002, Alborz 2005). These are some of the important issues which current service strategy – Health facilitation and Health Action Planning aim to address. World Health Organisation (2001 cited in Blackburn 1991) claimed that poor health status of people with learning disabilities is rooted in history of devaluation and exclusion in addition to other structural and environmental factors.

Chapter Two
Methodology

This dissertation uses qualitative methods, drawing on secondary data from available research studies and academic as well as practice discussions published in reputable journals. The author makes use of locally and nationally available data on *Valuing People* with regards to implementation of Health Facilitation and Health Action Planning as twin strategies for improving health of adults with learning disabilities from its inception in 2001 to the present time.

Aims of study

This dissertation aims to:

1. To explore the nature of health needs of people with learning disabilities.

2. To explore the concept of "health" and "health inequalities" in relation to this population.

3. To critically explore the definitions of Health Facilitation and Health Action Plan

4. To critically evaluate how Health Facilitation and Health Action Plan strategy is being implemented by the local Learning Disability Partnership Board.

5. To make recommendations regarding areas of good practice and or service gaps in the light of outcomes of this study.

To achieve these aims the method and sources used are

1. Extensive literature search and review.

2. Review and analyses where available of published national evaluation reports on the impact of *valuing people* in general and health outcomes for people with learning disabilities in particular.

3. Critically examines the local documents which set out local action plans to implement *Valuing People* health strategy.

4. Local Report on Independent evaluation of Health Action Plan

5. Evaluates local CLDT Business Plans 2003 – 2005, 2005 – 2007 with a view to determining service vision, direction and resource allocation in this respect.

6. Examines local health initiatives aimed at people with learning disabilities. Visit to neighbouring CLDTs to find out how these teams are implementing Health Facilitation and Health Action Planning in their areas.

7. Obtain and examine Action for Health Frameworks i.e. Health Action Plan and Health Facilitation strategy documents from different specialist learning disabilities teams in England. However, this will be limited to those freely available on these teams' web sites. See list of these teams in Appendix 1

Literature Review

Demonstrating reference to and use of existing body of knowledge is essential in the conduct of any research. Searching for what is already known on an area of study needs to be deliberate, systematic and rigorous. Hart (1998) described it as the selection of available published or unpublished documents on the subject matter capturing established facts and perceptions with a view to achieving some defined new study aims. Burns (2000) described it as "stimulus for thinking" and "sounding board" for new ideas p. 390. Literature review also needs to be explicitly stated to make the process of identifying, evaluating and interpreting the existing knowledge reproducible (Fink 1998).

Search Strategies

From the proposal stage of this dissertation the writer divided the subject matter into central themes reflecting the study questions. These themes were

- Trends in service provision for people with learning disabilities
- Health and health inequality in relation to people with learning disabilities
- Barriers to accessing same quality health care as other members of the population.
- Impact of *Valuing People* on current service provision for people with learning disabilities
- Health Facilitation for people with learning disabilities
- Health Action Planning for people with learning disabilities

The process of literature review can be divided into three stages (Finks 1998) which are: choosing key words, conducting the search and identifying relevant literature through established databases and manual bibliography search, clearly stating what criteria were used to include or exclude literature. The other two stages involved reading the literature and collecting data, and analysing and synthesising the key issues arising form those literature.

Key words used were '*Valuing people*', '*health facilitation*', '*health action planning*' '*health inequality and people with learning disabilities*'. However, learning disability as a key word presented with problem as this terminology is not universally accepted to refer to this population. The fact that the term is also used in education to refer to some specific learning difficulties such as dyslexia (Department of Health 2001) meant that much of the literature which the key word attracted were not relevant to the area of study. To capture international perspectives on the subject, alternative key words used were *mental handicap, mental retardation, cognitive and intellectual disabilities.*

Starting with London Metropolitan University Library, the writer first conducted manual searches of bibliography and subject index. Some useful text books especially on health inequality were found. However, search for books on learning disability yielded limited result and the few books found were all published before 2001. None of them were relevant to the central theme of this study i.e. implementation of Health facilitation and Health Action Planning. This problem may be due in part to the fact that the University does not offer any specialist course in Learning Disability. To circumvent this problem the writer used London Greenwich University Library which has a strong academic department on learning disabilities running courses such as Learning disability branch of nursing. Other libraries used were Royal College of Nursing and the King Fund. This helped the writer to locate up-to-date published books on the subject.

However, the bulk of the literature identified included journal and research articles published in reputable journals. Electronic databases proved invaluable in this regard. Those searched were British Nursing index, CINAHL (Cumulative index to Nursing Allied Health Literature) MEDLINE, PSYCINFO and King Fund. Access to these databases was gained through the London Metropolitan University and Health Information for London (HILO) which the writer gained access to through working in the NHS. The writer was denied access to some journals as London Metropolitan University did not subscribe to them. This double points of access to databases helped in gaining permission to wider journals. Even then, the writer was still denied access to some journals articles. Most of literatures obtained were free text of easily available full text articles.

In addition, the writer employed internet search engine such as Google, Google Scholar and Yahoo to find some additional preliminary and secondary sources. Though much of the information obtained through the link provided by these search engines were either grey literature which have not been published, these included personal opinions of writers, conference proceedings, reports, voluntary and statutory learning disability organisation web sites. Gray (2004) described grey literature as materials which may be published or unpublished that can not be identified through normal bibliographic methods. For instance, Mencap which is the largest charity organisation for people with learning disabilities in the UK has a good web site providing information and advice on the needs of people with learning disabilities and service provision in Britain. The writer used reference and bibliography of pages of selected literature as useful signpost to other relevant publications.

With regards to *Valuing People*, Health Facilitation and Health Action Planning policy implementation, the writer looked for literature that was written from 2001 – 2006. The literature must have in part or on the whole addressed the issue of health needs of people with learning disability and *Valuing People* must have been referenced. Though, other literature addressing issues such as housing and employment were scanned for possible relevance in relation to determinants of health and illness in this population.

In order to determine how the local CLDT initiatives compared with other similar areas, the writer visited and spent some time at three neighbouring

CLDTs in London. The writer discussed with some colleagues within these teams, including Health Facilitation Leads and some managers. The writer gathered information on how each of these teams was implementing Health Facilitation and Health Action Planning. Apart from obtaining copies of each of these team's Health Action Plan and Health Facilitation Frameworks, the writer was particularly interested to find out what specific decisions and initiatives have been taken around these strategies and also to find out about resource implications and challenges that these teams have experienced. The method of data gathering was informal, exploratory and shadowing to enable these colleagues to speak freely on the issues. The writer was conscious of ethical requirements when interviewing humans or employees in a research, but it was felt that in as much as the writer's contact with these teams was limited to networking and exploratory in which no individual would be quoted or referenced, an ethical clearance would not be required. The writer assured those professionals who spoke to him of confidentiality of their identities and none of the teams would be identified in this dissertation. Also, no client related clinical details are used in this study.

Chapter Three
A historical perspective of service provisions for people with learning disabilities

Care, treatment and support service provision for people with learning disabilities have taken different dimensions that are informed largely by the nature of historical landscapes along the way. Socio-economic and political realities influenced the way the society reacted and or responded to the need of this population. The present day status of people with learning disabilities and current philosophy of care and service provision can only be appreciated when juxtaposed with the past situation. This is not merely to glorify the progress made to date but to identify, where necessary, areas needing further developments.

Industrial period and the emergence of asylum

In the pre-industrial period, British society was essentially agrarian and the family units were the main means of production. People with learning disabilities lived with their families. Those whose learning disabilities were mild to moderate would also work on the farms to till the land and to attend to family live stocks. Mencap on its web site suggested that lack of good health care at that period meant that very few children with profound disabilities of any kind would survive beyond their early infancy. Some of the terminologies used to refer to this group of people included "village idiots" and "imbeciles". People with learning disabilities and those with mental health problems were seen more or less as the same and societal attitude towards them similar (Kelly 2000). Gilbert & Scragg (1992 cited in Gilbert 2003) catalogued other terminologies and phrases used to describe people with learning disabilities that were indicative of prevalent attitude towards them such as "mentally subnormal", "eternal child", "threat to society", "burden on society", "object of pity" and "sick". These terminologies had far reaching negative consequences on people with learning disabilities as they were by de facto accorded little or no rights.

With the industrial revolution and the collapse of subsistence farming, people with learning disabilities were seen as unproductive group which society needed to look after (Kelly 2000). They were segregated and shut away from society in large asylums and institution. For instance, the 1886 Idiot Act directed that local authorities should establish asylum for the care, education and training of the mentally disordered. The Act stated that 'idiots' do not include 'lunatics' thereby making attempt to distinguish learning disabilities from mental illness. The care of people with learning disabilities was at best paternalistic.

Another significant mile stones along the way included Mental Deficiency Act 1913 which defined "Mental Deficiency" and gave extensive power to hospital Board of Governors to detain and prevent discharge from the asylum of any inmate they deemed 'unfit' for release. People with learning disabilities were deemed to be incompetent to look after themselves, there was also belief that they were a threat to the society Gate (1997). Once someone was admitted to an institution on the ground of what the Act called "certified mental deficiency" discharge back into the community could take many years if at all. Local authorities were responsible for these asylums.

With the creation of the National Health Service (NHS) in 1948, care and treatment of people with learning disabilities became the responsibility of the NHS and the asylum became 'Hospital' culminating in whole adoption of a medical model of care. Apparently, there was no evidence that learning disability as a phenomena was curable, Yet, medical model of service provision meant that hospital based doctors had the overall care responsibility supported by qualified nurses trained in "mental sub normality".

Changing philosophy of care and the rise of new thinking

By 1950, the confinement of people with learning disabilities into hospital institutions had started to be challenged. This period set the stage for the eventual closure of those hospitals and the start of deliberate policy of resettling people back into the community. Damaging effects of institutionalisation on individuals began to be recognised and highlighted (Atherton 2000). By 1960, the Press had started to reveal catalogue of stories of serious abuses and neglect in these long stay hospitals. The impoverished and squalid living conditions, lack of privacy, physical mistreatment and abuse by staff had started to make headlines in Britain and these incidences had become subject of major public enquiries (Atherton 2005, Gilbert 2003 & Perini 2000). This period also witnessed the emergence of sociological studies that demonstrated that significant number of people with learning disabilities who were living in the institutions had the intellectual and social capabilities to live independently in the community (Atherton 2000). It should be pointed out that disability rights movement highlighting social and economic inequities faced by the disabled people as a whole had become more influential especially in the western industrialised countries (Barnes et al 1999). It was within this movement that campaign for better services for people with learning disabilities gained its incentive.

In 1971 the government released a White Paper entitled "Better services for the Mentally Handicapped" (Department of Health and Social Security 1971). The White Paper called for the closure of all the long stay hospitals, urging these facilities to set target dates for closure. This marked the beginning of intense activities towards a major policy shift by the government from custodial care to community care for people with learning disabilities in Britain. De-institutionalisation became official policy. Internationally, the United Nations in 1971 issued a Universal Declaration on the rights of the Mentally Retarded which articulated that people with learning disabilities had equal social, economic, health and political rights. The Declaration states that every individual with learning disabilities should receive appropriate support based on their needs to enjoy those rights.

Nationally, the White Paper *Better services for the mentally handicapped* (Department of Health and Social Security 1971) brought about an explosion in small community based residential care homes for people with learning disabilities. Long stay hospital had stopped taking new admissions and they were also discharging their residents back into the community.

The NHS and Community Care Act (1990) subsequently made it a legal requirement that people with learning disabilities and other vulnerable people should be provided with services based on assessed needs to enable them to live as normal life as possible. The Act conferred on the Social Services Department the lead agency status in planning, arranging and commissioning services for people with learning disabilities. This was as a result of recognition that the needs of people with learning disabilities were primarily social and not health. Though it was stressed that both agencies needed to work together to ensure that people are able to enjoy their social opportunities.

Meanwhile, some other powerful unofficial social policies in the forms of new concepts and philosophies which had direct impact in the way services were planned and delivered to this client group started to emerge. The most significant of these was *"Normalisation principles"* (Wolfenberger 1972). *Normalisation* was an extremely influential philosophy (Garner & Chapman 1993) which set out process of valuing positively individuals and groups who had been hitherto disvalued. The principle called for the society as a whole and generic health and social care services including specialist learning disabilities services to make concepts such as respect, and dignity, integration and participation rather than isolation and exclusion the cornerstone of their services. Normalisation was to have a profound impact on the direction of future services for this client group. O'Brien (1986 cited in Whitehead 1992) took normalisation principles further by coming up with his famous *'Five Service Accomplishments'* as a set of goals and standards on which services for people with learning disabilities must be based and measured. The five 'accomplishments' are Dignity and respect, Community presence and Community participation i.e. that people with learning disabilities should not only be assisted to live in the community they must be assisted to be active participants in the local communities. The other two areas are promoting Choice and Competence in all areas of daily activities.

These new principles provided people with learning disabilities, their carers and practitioners in this field a renewed focus, impetus and sound philosophical foundation to challenge mainstream services to provide inclusive services that address the individual needs of this population.

Previous attempts at addressing health needs of people with learning disabilities

However, while focus had been on social emancipation and integration of people with learning disabilities through provision of suitable and appropriate housing, day opportunities and practical support for them and their carers, it began to emerge that their health needs were not being met (Social Services Inspectorate 1998).

In response to new evidence that people with learning disabilities suffer more physical illness than the general population, between 1995 and 2001, government issued four official documents in the forms of good practice guidance and strategies highlighting not only the health issues and barriers faced by people with learning disabilities but also advising on how these health needs can be addressed. These documents are

The Health of the Nation: A strategy for people with learning disabilities (Department of Health 1995): This document acknowledged that adequate attention had not been paid to the health needs of this population. It states that many people with learning disabilities need help to choose a healthy way of life, to find out if they have an illness so that they can be treated, and to get help to access good health care if they become unwell. *Health of the Nation strategy for learning disabilities* however focused on five health issues namely; heart disease, cancer, sexual health, accidents and mental illness which were government priority areas for health promotion at the time. The Department of Health (1995) pointed out that people with learning disabilities have equal rights to all health promotion services such as health surveillance and health education, including unrestricted access to primary and secondary health care.

Signpost to Success (Department of Health 1998) was aimed primarily at service Commissioners and local health improvement programmes to ensure that people with learning disabilities get good quality services from the NHS. Signpost to Success is a non bidding "good practice guidance" document with the aim of helping local NHS especially the Primary Care teams to make their services more accessible to people with learning disabilities.

Once a Day (NHS executive 1999) was yet another good practice document in report form. It was aimed mainly at the GPs and other Primary Care teams. It aimed to promote good practice in enabling people with learning disabilities to access and receive good quality primary healthcare. To highlight the scale of the issue, the document's full title was a statement *"Once a day, one or more people with learning disabilities are likely to be in contact with your primary care team. How can you help them?"* It provided advice and guides on how to break the identified health barriers.

All these documents were part of government's efforts to get the message across to the whole NHS that people with learning disabilities represent a significant part of the population and that they are largely being excluded from services. That the NHS must work to improve the health experience of people with learning disabilities who use their services.

However, there is no evidence that these documents and government initiatives had any impact on the mainstream NHS. There is no nationally available data relating to mainstream health service experience of people with learning disabilities. Meanwhile, studies conducted by Bond et al (1997), Alborz et al (2004) and Disability Right Commission (2006) as well as anecdotal evidence from practice experience of the writer would suggest that why the documents provided learning disabilities specialist teams with increased ammunition and tools to challenge mainstream health care providers to provide better services to this population, it appeared that these mainstream services were often not aware of these documents. Perhaps more importantly is the empowerment which people with learning disabilities, their carers and those who work with them got through these documents which, one can argue laid foundation for *Valuing People*.

Chapter Four
Tackling health inequalities and improving the health of people with learning disabilities according to *Valuing People*

The progress made in learning disabilities service provision in the last 30 years has been described as revolutionary (Emerson 2005, Gilbert & Rose 1998). According to Mckenzie (2005), the medical model which assumes presence of disease in an individual which a doctor has the skills to diagnose and treat, is devaluing and an unhelpful way of responding to the needs of people with learning disabilities at micro and macro level. A social model of care which adopts holistic approach and sees health as being determined by many other factors such as environment, economic, psychological, social, cultural including biological factors is now the dominant approach. Yet, by 1999 it has become apparent that people with learning disabilities were still largely excluded from the mainstream of the society including the National Health Service. Mencap (1998) in its Report aptly titled "The NHS – Health for *all?*" argued that despite the gains of social model, rejection of medical model of care has resulted in the loss of focus on health needs of people with learning disabilities.

Why *Valuing People* White Paper?
It has been claimed that *Valuing People* is a direct result of failure of past rhetoric (Race 2002). While government acknowledged that the mainstream health services have failed people with learning disabilities as their services remained largely inaccessible to this population (DoH 2001), it has also been argued that specialist service provision for people with learning disabilities varied greatly across the country to the extent that consistency, quality and pattern were difficult to measure as there was no specified service goal

(Earwaker & Todd 1995). Hitherto learning disability service has never had a clear comprehensive national implementation strategy to ensure action across social and health needs of people with learning disabilities. Considering the population of people with learning disabilities in England as mentioned earlier, the need for a clear strategy became paramount and urgent. *Valuing People* can also be seen as continuation of the New Labour government modernisation agenda and a realisation that health and social care for vulnerable and disadvantaged people must take an integrated approach in which the root causes of health inequalities are targeted and addressed. It is a continuation of labour government's inclusion agenda that are emphasised across government departments. It is therefore not a coincidence that the new learning disability Strategy takes a holistic approach to meeting the needs of people with learning disabilities by laying out strategies for housing, work and leisure, support for carers and not just health, covering children and adults. This attempt to tackle, comprehensively, the inequality experienced by this population set the Strategy apart from previous attempts. However, the same comprehensiveness has attracted criticisms. McGill (2005) described *Valuing People* as complex as it tries to take on the impossible task of prescribing what needs to happen across all aspects of people with learning disabilities lives.

With regards to health, government modernisation objectives include improving access to primary and secondary health care and reducing inequities in the use of mainstream health services by disadvantaged and socially excluded section of the population (Alborz 2005). Government was determined to ensure that people with learning disabilities, like other sections of the population in England, receive health care service that is effective, appropriate and efficient (String & Grant 2005). However, it is acknowledged that people with learning disabilities would need deliberate and focused help to access and take full benefits of healthcare services. In this respect, Department of Health (2001) states that individual with learning disabilities would need a Health Facilitator who would help the individual challenge existing barriers and navigate the health service system. The Health Facilitators are also expected to assist individuals to develop and implement a Health Action Plan should the individual choose to have one.

Health Facilitation as a strategy to meet the health needs of people with learning disabilities

Collins New English Dictionary defined 'facilitate' as "to make easier" while in Blackwell's Dictionary of Nursing 'facilitation' is defined as "the act of increasing the ease with which an action or function is carried out". In this respect, what needs to be made easier for people with learning disabilities is the process of accessing appropriate healthcare when required. Introducing the concept of health facilitation and a designated individual to take on this role is an admission that people with learning disabilities largely lack the capacity to challenge the health inequalities which they experience. Whitehead (1992) observed that while service provision for this population has moved away from the medical model, they have only moved to an advocacy model involving other people to speak on behalf of disabled people. In this respect health facilitation can be seen as active health advocacy for and on behalf of a learning disabled person. Sanderson (2003) also described current service model as promotion of community membership, while Whitehead (1992 pp.371) described it as provision of "functional support" which may involve providing an individual with practical one-to-one support to attend medical and or leisure activities. *Valuing People* proposed that Health Facilitators will help people with learning disabilities access help, care and treatment they need to stay healthy. The White Paper classified Health facilitation into two levels tackling issues both at macro service level and at micro individual level. These two levels are referred to simply as level one and two:

Health facilitation at level two involves individual one-to-one support and it is expected that virtually anybody including parents, partners and friends who are close to the learning disabled person and not just specialist learning disability staff can take on this role. In this sense, the White Paper declared that "health facilitation *whoever does* it and in whatever way *in whatever setting* is about *ensuring healthier and better health* for people with learning disabilities" (DoH 2001 p. 12) (the italic emphases were writer's). Health facilitators are expected to assist in monitoring individual's health outcomes using the Health Action Plan framework. However, the assumption that "anybody can do it" is problematic. Turner (2001 p. 63) pointed out that "establishing an accurate and comprehensive picture of the physical health of people who have learning disabilities is a complex task". The nature of the individual health needs, especially in people who have profound and multiple learning and physical disabilities and the nature of learning disabilities itself may mean that health advocacy and facilitation would require high level of health awareness, good knowledge of locally available health facilities, good record keeping and high negotiation and assertive skills that many carers lack (Aborz 2005).

Though it is acknowledged that health facilitation evolved from traditional role of the family (Department of Health 2001), the Strategy failed to recognise other types of carers such as staff at residential care homes where many people live, and who have similarly supported their service users to access health care services. One can also argue that staff at Community teams, especially Learning Disability Nurses have always played leading roles in health advocacy for their clients through direct client works and indirect work with both primary and secondary health care services. Several studies (McCray & Carter 2002, McCray 2003, Barr 2004) and journal articles (Juke 2000, Jukes & Bollard 2002, & Parrish & Styring 2003) confirmed this point. Barr (2004) described the role of Learning disability Nurses as promoting and championing equity of access to health care services for people with learning disabilities, using their knowledge and skills to enable people with learning disabilities to exercise their right to the same quality of healthcare service as other valued citizens, including demanding extra resources, support and adaptation that may be required for such quality service to be provided. McCray (2003) in a study which explored the roles of learning disability nurses within a multidisciplinary setting reported that learning disability nurses are used to coordinating care of people with learning disabilities, and that they have clearer understanding of other professionals' role . Learning Disability Nurses have a more holistic approach to health facilitation (Lindsey 2002) and they had been taking leading roles both at level one (Strategic) and level two (direct client work) health facilitation. It is in this recognition that the Department of Health (2001) stated that Learning disability Nurses are "best placed" to take on health facilitation role, while at the same time inviting other professionals within the Community Learning disabilities team to take on the role. In this sense, one can actually say that Health Facilitation at this level is nothing new. Perhaps what is new is the proposal that all professionals within the CLDT must now include health facilitation as part of their roles, therefore moving away from traditional assumption that this a role only for learning disability nurses. However, the Department of Health (2001) realized that learning disability nurses are in short supply and would not be able to cope with the volume of work that the new initiatives were sure to generate. For instance, Flynn (2002) observed that nationally there are 11,000 learning disability nurses against estimated 1.2 million people with learning disability. This was also against the background that every learning disabled individual was expected to have a "clearly identified" allocated person as his or her Health Facilitator by June 2003 (DoH 2001). Three years after this target date, it remains unclear how well health facilitation role has been received by other health specialities. The writer did not come across any research or evaluation that have reviewed or studied either resource implication of health facilitation and or how well other professionals within specialist learning disabilities teams have incorporated this into their roles. However, Alborz et al (2003) in their literature review on access to health care for people with learning disabilities reported that having a health facilitator is effective in identifying undiagnosed conditions, raising awareness and generating solutions in addition to communicative and liaison utility of the approach.

Meanwhile *Valuing People* recognizes that tackling health inequalities in this respect is beyond individual one-to-one health facilitation work. It proposes that there must be parallel broader strategy at macro level that will involve development work targeting mainstream services to make their services more accessible to people with learning disabilities. Level One Health Facilitation involves development works with mainstream health services as well as close proactive and collaborative work with these services, offering their staff training and advice on learning disabilities. It involves working with the GPs to identify people with learning disabilities on their register with a view to offering them appropriate health surveillance such as routine health screening and required treatments. *Valuing People* proposed that each Community Learning Disabilities Team should identify someone to take on this strategic health facilitation lead role. Again, there has not been any national data that has demonstrated the effectiveness of having a designated lead person in this regards, though, there appear to be some consensus in learning disability services that having someone who focuses on building bridge across specialist learning disability services and mainstream health services would not only raise the profile of health needs of people with learning disabilities but also help them to get better services. Williamson (2004) argued that health facilitation is slower, harder to manage, and at times, frustrating, a strategic approach is more likely to reduce inequalities, challenge discrimination and raise service quality for all members of the population. Examples of this are found in some areas across the country where Health Facilitation Lead is working with the GPs in their areas to ensure that every learning disabled person on the team's register is offered an annual health check which one-to-one health facilitators or other designated persons can then support the client to attend. Some of these teams have also developed health questionnaires which are then administered by a GP as part of annual health check. This is a direct result of mounting research evidence that clearly showed that people with learning disabilities miss out on many health surveillance activities and that regular health checks do help to identify new unmet health needs (Alborz 2005).

Strategic Health Facilitation should also include offering Primary care staff training in learning disabilities. Russell (2006) reported on a project in which a health resource pack was developed with the help of people with Down Syndrome to raise GPs awareness of issues concerning this clients group. Russell (2006) claimed that lack of understanding of learning disabilities by GPs for instance, in addition to their difficulties in communicating with people with learning disabilities can leave the GPs feeling unskilled and that significant number would consider withdrawing their services from this population or alternatively demand extra pay for treating patients with a learning disability. The issue of offering the GPs monetary incentive is controversial as it can be argued that as equal member of the society, people with learning disabilities are by right entitled to a decent health care like anybody else.

Health facilitation at level 1 therefore takes a long term strategic approach to develop the infrastructure to support inclusion. Other activities may involve working with acute hospitals to adopt a person centred approach in their admission and discharge process for people with learning disabilities and advising the hospitals on how to make their information leaflets, communication medium and systems accessible to this population. From some Health Facilitation Frameworks and Strategy documents which the writer obtained and analysed, it was evident that many teams across the country have appointed a designated learning disability nurse as Access to Acute Liaison Nurse (A2A) to tackle problem of access to general hospitals for people with learning disabilities.

Health Action Plan: as a tool to make things happen

The corner stone principle in *Valuing People* is Person Centred Planning. *Valuing People* stipulates that all services for people with learning disabilities must demonstrably adopt this approach in the process of commissioning, planning and delivery of services. Many literatures referred to Health Action Planning as "Person Centred Health Action Planning" to highlight the fact that the most important consideration in the process of helping individual to live healthy life is the individual. DoH (2001) defined Health Action Plan as a personal plan which details necessary actions which an individual needs to take to maintain and improve his or her health, including the help the individual would need to successfully carry out those necessary actions. In its "Good Practice Guidance" (DoH 2002) described it as a mechanism that will help link individual with appropriate services. It was anticipated that Health Action Plan would be helpful in educating and informing individual learning disabled person about their health and to help service coordination by individual's Health Facilitator. A Health Action Plan is simply a personal health record. It focuses on individual health issues in a deliberate and structured way by identifying and addressing issues such as the health needs of the individual and stating actions that are necessary to address the needs. It also addresses who will take what action, the time limit for each action to be taken, mechanism to monitor and evaluate progress. The plan will also detail other important information about the individual such as their medications and the preferred method of communication see *Five Questions of Health Action Plan* on pg 62. Each area is expected to put in place a clear strategy on how Health Action Plan will be delivered. In this respect, many CLDT in England have developed different tools to be used as individual potable personal health needs and action record. Consequently, the name, contents, scope, accessibility and designs varied greatly from team to team. In the local area of study the tool is called "My Health Matters". It is called "Personal Health Profile" in another area.

Evidence to back the impact of Health Action Plan is scarce. However, Burchell & Turk (2003) and Howatson (2005) claimed that the idea of hand-held health records is not new. What is new is rolling this out across England. Burchell & Turks (2003) likened Health Action Plan to type of hand held health record widely used in maternity and children services and other specialist services for some medical conditions such as diabetes. In their literature review on Health Action Plan, Burchell and Turks (2003) reported that while there is no concrete evidence that having a personal health record brings about a better health outcome for the individuals, many people with learning disabilities reported that they found the tool useful in communicating their needs to other people and that they feel more empowered using it. This is consistent with findings by Pratt et al (2005) in the evaluation of local Health Action Plan tool pilot where parents of some people with learning disabilities also said that they found the tool as effective communicative tool and at the same time helping them to remember and focus on important health issue for their sons or daughters during GP and other health appointments. Pratt et al (2005) also found out that Health Action Plan tool helped in identifying additional areas of health needs in clients who participated in the pilot. Yet there is no concrete evidence that identifying new health needs necessarily lead to subsequent prompt and effective treatments and or services for individual concerned. Martin et al (2004) also claimed that Health Action Plan helps update individual heath records and helps the individual to be better understood by professionals other than those who are already familiar with their needs.

However, Young & Chesson (2006) observed that the evidence base with regards to outcomes of health intervention in people with learning disabilities is weak, perhaps due to the fact that outcome measure in health is embedded in the quantitative approach to the extent that for instance we can determine how many more people with learning disabilities receive medical screenings. Or how many people received as a result of their Health Action Plan better diabetes specialist services. One could also argue that strictly speaking, a personal health record is neither a valid nor reliable health needs assessment tool as it depends hugely on the ability of the individual with learning disabilities to disclose necessary health information and the ability of the helper to elicit and record this information. It also depends on level of cooperation from primary as well as acute care staff including the GP and appropriate Specialists who are involved in the individual's care and treatments.

Another criticism is that there is real danger of Health Action Plan degenerating into elaborate paper activity which if not managed carefully could lead to unnecessary duplication of people's health information without any commensurate positive health outcome. Person Centred Plan, Health Facilitation and Health Action Plan are themselves not accessible terminologies that can be easily understood by people with learning disabilities who these initiatives are meant to serve. One can then argue that these terminologies may further disempowered people with learning disabilities as they rely on other people especially professionals to explain what these meant. Despite the controversy surrounding the effectiveness of both Health facilitation and Health Action Plan they appeared to have been well received within learning disability services in the country.

Chapter Five

Strategic actions for health: A local implementation of Health Facilitation and Health Action Planning

It is argued that for any organisation to be successful its action must be determined by clear strategic plan which takes accounts of all important environmental factors. The local Community Team for People with Learning Disabilities is no exception to this. Its objectives, priorities, policies and programmes must not only match its service users' expectation, but also those of its stakeholders. Strategy has been defined as "the match an organisation makes between its internal resources and the threat and opportunities created by the external environment in which it operates" (Bowan & Asch1987 cited in Lawton 1999 p. 121).

Valuing People did not impose any process of implementation on local areas, but it leaves organisations to take into account local situations and needs. Before embarking on any change process or developing a local strategy, it is important for organisations to have a good understanding of the environment in which they operate. From its Health Action Plan Framework, it would appear that the Partnership Board carried out what appeared to be a good analysis of its situation prior to implementation of Health Action Planning and Health facilitation. While it is unclear which model of environmental analysis was used by the team, the document lists what it referred to as its strengths and weaknesses and tried to anticipate challenges in the implementation of *Valuing People* health agenda in the local area. Outhwaite (2003) advised that a situational analysis is an essential part within any process of change and it is actually the starting point for forming strategy as it helps in considering various factors impacting on service development. Fyson & Ward (2004) also argued that strategic planning needs to be based on accurate information not only on targeted population but also existing services and unmet needs. It would also appear from the Framework that relevant stakeholders were clearly identified and the process of consultation made clear.

Valuing People health agenda is anchored on four principles of *right, choice, participation* and *inclusion*. It is about mainstreaming the health needs of people with learning disabilities and this requires statutory and voluntary organisations to work together in a way they had never done before. The local CLDT and the Partnership Board quickly recognised that all partnership organisations – local NHS and social care service providers in particular would need to demonstrate their commitment to meeting the health needs of people with learning disabilities in the area. The process of achieving collaborative working and good working relationship among local organisations required identifying existing good practices, development of new initiatives, and new ways of working and new resources.

Also, at the inception of *Valuing People* a joint service integrating Community Health Team for people with learning disabilities and Social Services Adult Community Team for people with learning disabilities was being developed. A review of both teams was also taking place involving management process, arrangements for care management, single point of entry system, single assessment process and care co-ordination. Locally there was no register for people with learning disabilities hence there was no reliable statistics on which to base service plan. It was unclear how many people were on the CLDT case load, this was coupled with the fact that there was little understanding of the expectations arising from Health Action Planning and Health Facilitation proposal. The period was therefore a particularly anxiety provoking one for all concerned. This was against the background of other far reaching modernisation and inclusion agenda that was taking place within the NHS.

Local Context

The 2001 Census puts the population of this London Borough at 243,737. Cole (2006) in a recent survey report commissioned by Learning Disability Partnership Board estimated the population as at mid 2004 to be 247,700 people. Using audit tool and *Valuing People* assumption that 25 people out of every 1000 will have mild to moderate learning disabilities, 4 people in 1000 will have severe learning disabilities; Cole (2006) estimated that out of the total population 7,183 people have learning disabilities. Out of this figure, 6,192 local people will have mild to moderate learning disabilities and 991local people are expected to have severe learning disabilities. Most of these people will require extensive support in many areas of daily living. 50% of local people with moderate to severe learning disabilities are estimated to also have some additional physical or sensory impairment, while 25% have mental health support needs (Learning Disability Health Task Group 2003). Community Learning disabilities team has on its newly developed register 1,222 adults with varying degrees of abilities and needs.

This area of London is one of the most deprived boroughs in London and poverty is real issue. According to Learning Disability Health Task Group (2003), the increasing number of young people with learning disabilities in the local community places added strain on local services, with estimated 29 babies with severe learning disabilities born in the area every year. It is unclear how this figures compared with other areas of London.

The borough has a very diverse population with 60.6% of the population from black and ethnic minority communities. 32% of this is from south Asian community. According to Hatton et al (1997 cited in Pratt et al 2005) the prevalence of learning disabilities is higher in this population.

Actions for Health: Vision and expectations

The implication of *Valuing People* as a strategy is that no two areas implement Health Facilitation and Health Action Plan in exactly the same way. This also became apparent from analysis of various local Health Action Plan Frameworks obtained for this work.

In line with *Valuing People* the local strategy aimed to achieve targets set in the *Valuing People* with the overall aim of bringing about a "systematic change necessary to improve the health of people with learning disabilities, and sustain this over time", pp. 10

This is located within a broad vision to make the local area:

> ... *a place where people with learning disabilities, whatever their level of need, have the same access as the rest of the community for social, educational and employment opportunities. This includes equal access to health care and leisure interests, and people having support appropriate to their culture and identity*

The framework stressed that all stakeholders would share responsibility for ensuring that people with learning disabilities can access mainstream health services and that they must all work for health promotion among their people with learning disabilities. While adopting the position of "it is everybody's job", the Learning Disabilities Partnership Board in the study area sets out clearly in a Framework its vision for learning disabilities service in general and it puts forward an action plan for achieving *Valuing People* health targets locally.

Declaration of vision, expectations, commitment and what needs to happen are not enough, how to deliver them is more important. Fyson (2005) argued that in many instances across the country local action plans often resembled ill defined wish list rather than coherent strategies that can achieve measurable objectives within specified framework. The next section takes a look at how *Valuing People* health agenda is being implemented in the area of study.

Initiatives to facilitate access to health care for local people with learning disabilities

Locally, Community Nurses for people with Learning disabilities have traditionally been responsible for supporting adults with learning disabilities who live in the community and whose social and health circumstances were such that they lack necessary ability and or support to access appropriate health care themselves. As pointed out earlier, several studies (McCray & Carter 2002, McCray 2003, Barr 2004) and journal articles (Jukes 2002, and Parrish & Styring 2003) have highlighted the roles of registered nurses who are trained in learning disabilities. McCray & Janet (2002) in another survey of carers found that Learning Disability Nurses received highest praise from parents and the study also found that they have credibility with other carers and professionals.

Locally available Nursing establishment simply would not be able to cope with the demands of Health Facilitation and Health Action Planning within this service. With eight full-time Community Nurses for people with learning disabilities in post, it is unrealistic to cover 1,222 clients on the Community Team's case load, let alone the whole learning disability population of 7183 in the case study as the White Paper implied. Community Learning Disabilities Nurses case load is primarily around individuals who had difficulties in accessing specific health care service, either through lack of appropriate support or complexity of the clients' health and or nature of their learning disabilities. Also while other professionals such as Physiotherapists, Psychologists, Speech and Language Therapists and Occupational Therapists undertake some basic health advocacy contacting GP for specific issues on behalf of their clients and or making onward referral to appropriate health services and following this through, it is only Community Nurses who provide these clients with both one-to-one nursing support helping them to arrange appointments, and if required, physically supporting these clients at appointments including in the case of hospital investigations or treatment, working with the clients and their carers and the hospital staff to ensure that the clients get maximum benefit from their hospital encounter.

Setting up a Working Group

At the inception of *Valuing People*, a Learning Disability Health Task Group was set up by the local Learning Disabilities Partnership Board comprising a broad representation from key stakeholders such as service users' groups (Men Group and Women group), Mencap, local Patient Advisory Liaison service (PAL), Carers' Network, Public Health, residential and day opportunity service prodders, Commissioning Manager and Specialist

Learning Disability professionals. This group met and put together the implementation strategy document mentioned above. The framework represented a broad consensus on strategies to ensure that health needs of local people with learning disabilities are addressed. Outhwaite (2003) argued that it is the local interpretation of *Valuing People* that is the most significant factor in relation to determining what types of services and collaborations that would be required. Through the Task Group the expectation that all local service providers would take responsibility for their role in ensuring the health needs of people with learning disabilities are identified and addressed received broad support. Pratt et al (2005) in their evaluation of the CLDT Health Action Planning Pilot reported that Health Action planning in the area has been informed by the views of people with learning disabilities and their carers through series of community based meetings and workshops organised by the Task Group. The Task Group offered a forum for discussing issues of importance with regards to health needs of local people with learning disabilities in general and the implementation of Health Action Plans in particular.

Developing a template for Health Actions

In line with the Department of Health good practice Guidance (2002) that each area should develop its own format/template for individual Health Action Plans. An accessible tool called *My Health Matters* was developed by the CLDT. Drawing from the advice and input from people with learning disabilities themselves, plain English, extensive photographs and symbols were used in the tool. After the tool was piloted and evaluated, it was rolled out across the Borough. A well attended workshop (Pratt et al 2005) was also held for the stakeholders on Health Action Planning and the tool. Issues that were raised at the workshop and the outcomes of the pilot evaluation were incorporated into the final tool.

However, the proposal that everyone with learning disabilities should be offered a Health Action Plan by June 2003 presented the Health Task Group a big challenge. In fact the team had to push the date forward to June 2005 as this date was deemed to be more realistic. One of the ways the problem was addressed was that the Health Task Group organised a health fair using the same title as the Health Action Plan tool for the event. The event which was widely publicised in the borough was jointly funded by the local Primary Care Trust and Social Services. The aim of the event was, among others, to raise the awareness of people with learning disabilities, their carers, learning disabilities and mainstream service providers to how Health Action Plan can help in meeting the health needs of local people with learning disabilities and to raise the profile of health needs of people with learning disabilities among the mainstream health care providers. The event was hailed by the local Press as a huge success. Between 350 and 400 people with learning disabilities and their carers attended the event. 31 mainstream health care providers from Primary Care to Acute secondary health care providers were represented at the event. Workshops on Health Action Plans were held throughout the day. And 450 copies of Health Action Plan tools were distributed on the day. An easy to understand process of getting help and assistance with putting together a Health Action Plans was highlighted and other accessible information leaflets such as tips on how to get good service from a GP was also distributed on the day. This is in response to the evidence Mackean (1999) that many people with learning disabilities experience anxiety when going to doctor's appointment which can disrupt and compromise the process of consultation

Appointing a Change Agent

Another significant step that was taken was the appointment of a Senior Community Learning Disability Nurse to the role of Health Facilitation Lead. This person acted as the change agent who provided the necessary leadership and direction for the initiatives. This role was strategic across the borough, taking a long term approach to tackling barriers to accessing health care services for local people with learning disabilities. The Health Facilitation Lead was responsible for co-ordinating the overall implementation of the Health Facilitation and Health Action Planning, working in partnership with people with learning disabilities, care service providers and specialist professional colleague within the CLDT. The role also included ensuring that the locally developed Health Action Plan tool was widely publicised, available and implemented throughout the borough including training individuals and carers to use the tool. At the time of this study (September 2006) 120 people comprising of carers in residential services, day opportunity centres, and Outreach support staff were reported to have been trained. The aim was that these paid carers would feel empowered and confident to support their clients to access appropriate mainstream health care services and also to help them to develop individual Health Action Plan. The Health Facilitation Lead was expected to ensure that Health Facilitation and Health Action Plan become an integral part of the individual Person Centred Plan (PCP) by working together with PCP facilitators in this regards. This post also built strong relationship with Patients and Public Involvement team and Patient Advisory Liaison team of the local hospitals and Primary Care Trust.

Facilitating access to Acute General Hospitals

Another initiative was an Access to Acute Healthcare Services project (A2A) which was developed to improve the experience of people with learning disabilities accessing general hospital services. The project received active support and input from the local NHS Patient Involvement Manager, Learning Disabilities Nurse Manager and service user's groups. An initially part-time Access-to-Acute Liaison Nurse was appointed to work with local general hospitals to ensure that these hospitals become more accessible for people with learning disabilities. Some of the activities in this project included establishing a protocol for admission and discharge of patients with learning disabilities, working with the hospitals to produce accessible information leaflets for patients with learning disabilities and working directly with patients and carers to ensure that the patients receive appropriate health care from the hospital that is sensitive to their needs. Work undertaken in this area was highly commended in the North East London Strategic Health Authority Modernisation Award for 2003 under the category of improving Access to services (Learning Disability Task Group 2003). The post subsequently became a full-time permanent one.

Facilitating access to mental health care

With regards to the mental health needs of people with learning disabilities, there is wide acceptance that people with learning disabilities have higher mental health problems (Gravestock & Bouras 1997) The Royal College of Psychiatrists (2003) argued that mainstream mental health services lack the skills, expertise and resources to manage people who have dual needs of learning disabilities and mental health problems. The College recommends intensive case management and collaborative approaches in this respect.

There is also evidence (Bouras & Holt 2000) that good inter-agency working and communication is crucial to meeting the needs of this group. *Valuing People* clearly states that the National Service Frame Work for mental health which was published in England by DoH in 1999 equally applies to people with learning disabilities and that effort should be made to ensure that people with learning disabilities are supported to access mainstream mental health services. In this regards a multi-agency mental health Liaison Group was set up to meet quarterly to promote joint working between the local CLDT and mental health team. A full-time Mental Health and Learning Disability Liaison Nurse post was also developed to facilitate access to all ranges of mental health services for people with learning disabilities who also experience mental health problems. This post combined level one strategic health facilitation with level two one-to-one clinical client works. The Liaison Nurse from time to time provides support, advice and training to mental health staff and carers.

Providing extra support to people with learning disabilities and their families

An outreach CLDT support service (Intensive Support Service) that provides some one-to-one practical support to individual with learning disabilities to enable them to take full benefit of health care services was set up. Though, this initiative predated *Valuing People* as it has been in existence since 1996, it wholly met the proposal in the White Paper that local specialist community services across the country should consider setting up an "Intensive Health Care Support" (DoH 2001 p. 69) that would provide sensitive support tailored to individual needs. The local service helps people whose social circumstances are such that they do not have adequate support and there is a risk that their health could deteriorate as a result. For instance people who live on their own or with elderly carers who may have health needs of their own. The service would provide an experienced learning disability Care Assistant to support individuals at GP clinics, hospital appointments or to attend leisure or community activities that could enhance the health of the individual as part of care intervention strategy. An important area of this service also includes providing one-to-one staff support for people with learning disabilities who are on admission and undergoing treatment in hospital but who, due to the nature or manifestation of their learning disabilities, are at the risk of not getting full benefit from the hospital treatment or whose behaviour may disrupt their or other people's treatment. This service also enables parents and carers (especially elderly carers who may have health needs of their own) of the individual on admission to take a break from their caring role knowing that an experienced learning disability support staff is staying with their son or daughter. Nocon & Qureshi (1996) pointed out that caring can have serious negative impact on many areas of carer's lives such as mental and physical health as well as loss of earning. This is also in line with some of the evidence (Lindsey 2002, Bond et al (1997) highlighted earlier in this dissertation that mainstream staffs lack the knowledge, skill, attitude and patience to meet the health needs of this population.

Meeting the targets: barriers and challenges

Health Facilitation and Health Action planning was proposed at a time when there was a lot of confusion and anxiety in the air with regards to the process of integrating the local health and Social Services teams as a result of national health and social care reforms. At the time there was no clear line of command as the post of Joint Service Manager and Assistant Joint Service

Manager posts were vacant for about one year . Line of command was blurred with each head of disciplines sharing management responsibilities as an interim arrangement. This was in many cases in addition to their clinical and discipline specific management responsibilities. A clear and strong leadership would have helped to rally the staff together towards the implementation of *Valuing people* agenda and targets. Heller & Hindle (1998) pointed out that for a team to be successful it needs strong effective leadership that would initiate precise organisational objectives, take quick decisions on project at hand and communicate these freely to the team. The implication of the absence of leadership was that though local strategies for the implementation of Health Facilitation and Health Action Planning was in place many specific targets around Health Action Planning were delayed as necessary authority required for resources allocation in this regards was not available. Mullins (2005) argued that authority vested in a manager accords responsibility for staffing, and for the motivation and guidance of subordinates.

Health facilitation is about demanding change and inclusive healthcare services. It is about challenging mainstream health services to make reasonable adjustments to accommodate the health needs of people with learning disabilities. According to Jukes (2002), it also involves an effective management of change across professional boundaries as all health professionals in specialist learning disability services are expected to play a role.

Hitherto, disciplines except Community Learning Disability Nursing work, strictly on clinical episode of care. Understandably, there was resistance to the proposed change as some people believed that taking on level two one-to-one Health facilitation and Health Action plan roles would bring about an increase in their workload and distract them from their traditional clinical works. This situation is consistent with Mullin (2005) assertion that despite potential positive outcomes of change, it is often resisted at both individual and organisational levels. Nothing much has changed in this area as health facilitation continued to be seen as a nurse's job. Many clients therefore are yet to have an identifiable Health Facilitator and are yet to be offered Health Action Plans. This was further compounded by recruitment problems across disciplines, with some posts remaining vacant for up to one year. However, many people in residential homes and or Day opportunity Centres now have allocated health facilitators from within those organisation.

Despite these challenges it would appear that much mileage has been covered by the local CLDT. The team's business plan 2006 – 2007 contained an evaluation and assessment of achievements and progress up to date.

Integration of health and social care is now complete and clear management is now in place this has enabled the team to be more focused and motivated. A database of people with learning disabilities on the team's case load has now been set up and all people with learning disabilities known to the team are now registered with a GP in line with *Valuing People* priority. At the time of this dissertation a Reed code to enable local GPs to identify all patients with learning disabilities on their registered has just been agreed with the local PCT. A proposal has also been submitted to develop an Enhanced GP Service for people with learning disabilities under the New GP Contract Commissioning arrangement. Through the scheme GP would be paid extra money for providing extended and comprehensive services such as annual health check, completing Health Action Plans and hosting specific nurse lead health clinics. The team also developed a very successful "Special Parenting Project" which identified and supported parents who have learning disabilities to receive ante-natal and post-natal care. The project which comprised of a Community Learning Disability Nurse and two Clinical Psychologists did not only support expecting mothers with learning disabilities to access appropriate ante-natal health services, it also helped them by enhancing their parenting skills and thereby increased their chance of keeping their babies after birth. The project worked with all relevant agencies to minimize the risk of child protection procedure which many people with learning disabilities often experience. A Borough wide Protocol was developed. However, the project was funded for two years only.

Area of study vs other areas: a comparative analysis

Very little has been done to evaluate the impact of Health Facilitation and Health Action Plan nationally. Hatton et al (2005) pointed out that despite *valuing People* being around since 2001, national information to evaluate its objectives was yet to be available as at early 2005, making any evaluation of progress since the introduction difficult. However, Valuing People Support Team a body which is based at the Department of Health and is responsible for monitoring and providing guidance on the implementation of the White Paper published a report titled "Valuing People: the story so far" in March 2005" at about the same time Hatton et al made their comments. The report acknowledged what it called "some excellent work" being done "by some local people" to try and get the mainstream health services to address health inequalities and that "some general hospitals are making things better for people when they go into hospital" p. 17. However, the Report contained no hard fact on any aspect of *Valuing People* objective and there was no mention of Health Facilitation or Health Action Plan at all. It then becomes difficult to compare one area with the other.

However, in order to get an idea of what is happening somewhere else the writer obtained Health Action Plan Strategy Frameworks from three neighbouring CLDTs and the writer also networked and visited these teams to find out about how they are implementing Health Facilitation and Health Action Plan in their areas. One thing that was striking was how different each of these teams is in it approaches and identified priorities. While none of these teams has Access to Acute Liaison Nurse, Mental Health and Learning Disabilities Liaison Nurse nor anything equivalent to Intensive support Service and Special Parenting Project as in the area of study, one CLDT has secured Enhanced GP Service under the new GMS contract which came into effect in April 2004. It should be pointed out that under the new contract system, PCT are allowed to commission Enhanced GP Services to meet services addressing specific local health needs or innovative services (see detail on www.bma.org.uk/ap.nsf/content/focusenhanced0104). In this particular area 8 local GP practices were said to have signed up to provide enhanced services to local people with learning disabilities. These GPs are paid for extra work they provide around Health Action planning and annual health checks for each individual. Another CLDT secured a research grant from the Department of Health to evaluate local Health Action Plan tool. About 53 GP practices in the area who are participating in the research agreed to complete Health Action Plans for patients with learning disabilities on their register and also do follow up annual health check for them. In both CLDT the Health Facilitation Lead person worked closely with these Practice

Surgeries to identify each person with learning disabilities on GP register thereby meeting a vital *Valuing People* objective. The two neighbouring teams appeared to have made contact with and developed better working relationship with majority of local GP Practices. In both cases extra funding appeared to have accounted for this progress.

However, only one team has a clear strategy on Health Facilitation and Health Action Planning with regards to young people in transition from children to adulthood i.e. 16 – 18 years old. People with learning disabilities in this category are identified as a priority area in *Valuing People*. Using *neighbourhood renewal* funding the local team in question appointed separate Health Facilitation Lead for this group apart from the one for the older adults. According to Caan et al (2005) in their evaluation of Health facilitation in this particular CLDT the writer found that this post helped to improve the quality of transition plans for school leavers who were about to move to adult services.

As it was left to local services to introduce health facilitation either by extension of existing roles or by creation of new specialist posts (Caan 2005), in one CLDT a full time Health Facilitation Coordinator was in post, in the other two CLDTs including the area of study a Senior Community Learning Disability Nurse combined Health facilitation Lead role with clinical case work. Only one area has carried out an evaluation of the impact of Health Facilitation and or Health Action Plan on people with learning disabilities in its areas. Even in this team the evaluation was limited to only young people in transition. None of these teams has audited the uptake of Health Action Plan in its area. Hence, it was not clear how many people actually have Health Action Plans or allocated Health Facilitators. It therefore remains unclear what the impact of having a Health Facilitator and or Health Action Plan is on the individual health outcomes. As in the area of study, the writer found that in the neighbouring CLDTs, Health Facilitation is still largely left to Community Learning Disability Nurses and that *Valuing People*'s proposal that other professionals within the team should also take on these roles has not had any significant impact.

Conclusion and recommendations

As it has been shown in this work, while the status and profile of people with learning disabilities have improved over the last three decades, especially with regards to their community integration and social needs, they continue to experience barriers when accessing health care services. It is widely acknowledged that people with learning disabilities have poorer health and they are often left out of preventive health screening and health promotion activities. Negative attitude of health professionals, lack of knowledge and understanding of learning disabilities on the part of these health care workers, complex health service environment as well as communication difficulties which many people with learning disabilities have including the nature of individual's disabilities have been blamed.

Based on the principles of *right, choice, participation* and *inclusion, Valuing People* aimed to ensure that people with learning disabilities receive the same quality of health and social care as everyone else. It is acknowledged that people with learning disabilities would need planned and systematic help if they were to take full benefit of available health services, especially the NHS. Health Facilitation and Health Action Planning are suggested as ways of improving the health of this population.

As it has been shown in this work there is wide variation across England in the way Health Facilitation and Health Action Planning are being implemented and it is difficult to compare one area with the other. This is rather interesting development considering the fact that one of the stated reasons for *Valuing People* was the need to harmonise service provision for this client group across the country. From implementation strategy documents analysed for this dissertation, there appears to be a wide divergence with regards to the *input* i.e. number of dedicated specialist staff e.g. Health Facilitation Lead and Liaison Nurses created and the actual implementation *process* i.e. types of health initiatives such as health screening or health promotion activities as well as the nature of support system available for people with learning disabilities within each team. While some areas have invested huge time and financial resources to attract local GPs to provide patients with learning disabilities with extra consultation time, annual health screenings and input into individual Health Action Plans by commissioning Enhanced GP Services, some other areas have focused on close liaison work with acute secondary health care providers including mental health teams. There is no evidence to establish which of these implementation models is most effective with regards to bringing about the most important thing i.e. positive health *outcomes* for individuals with learning disabilities.

This writer is of the views that since the fast majority of people with learning disabilities now either live at home with their families or in other types of accommodations outside the NHS including shared residential and supported living, Specialist Learning Disabilities teams should target carers in these settings, offering them trainings specifically on health advocacy for people with learning disabilities. The Health Facilitation Lead within the local CLDT should also serve as a resource for consultation on Health Action Planning and how this can be integrated into any existing individual Person Centred Plan. The frontline staff and carers who have closet relationship with the individuals with learning disabilities are best placed to support them to access required health care services and these carers would need support and advice from the specialist learning disabilities professionals, especially from the Specialist Community Learning Disability Nurses. However, where an individual has unmet complex and multiple health needs or where individual's social circumstances e.g. those who live on their own, is such that he/she is at higher risk of unmet health needs, a system should be put in place that would make the case a priority allocation for the Specialist Community Learning Disability Nurses. Ultimately, quality of support that is at the disposal of an individual with learning disability is crucial to how effectively any barrier to accessing good healthcare would be challenged.

Post Scripts

- Five questions of Health Action Planning
- Common Health issues in people with learning disabilities and relevant health professionals
- Community Learning Disabilities Teams
- Qualities of a Health Facilitator
- Who can be a Health Facilitator?
- Consent and Mental Capacity

There is no rigid rule governing the format of a Health Action Plan. Templates and formats in use are as many and varied as learning disabilities team across England. What is important however is that any format adopted must be as relevant, individualised and accessible for the individual who owns the plan. However, this writer would argue that where an individual has profound and multiple cognitive disabilities, Health Action Plan can be of ordinary format which that individual's Health Facilitator and significant others can use on his/her behalf. In all cases there must be effort made and evidence shown to demonstrate client's involvement.

At the minimum, a Health Action Plan must address the following questions:

1. What are the health needs? (i.e. issues)

An up-to-date comprehensive Annual Health Check must have been carried out by the GP and the outcome fed into the Health Action Plan. With Client's permission, write to the GP and other health professionals involved in the client's care requesting for an up-to-date medical history. Add this information to what the clients and other significant others tell you and what you already know about the client's health. State the health issues clearly. Ask the GP to write treatment plans for any specific health issues including any on-going or clinical investigations or planned referral to any other specialist.

2. What actions are needed to address these identified health issues?

Identify what services are required for each of the health issues e.g. diabetes GP, Diabetes Specialist Nurse, Epilepsy – GP, Neurologist, Epilepsy Specialist Nurse etc. Identify what the client also needs to do including any life style changes. State what medications are prescribed and the level of support the client needs to take the medications, including how these would be monitored and reviewed.

3. Who will do what? (e.g. clients, carers, Key worker,

professionals, but who?). Does the client need specialist referral and who will make this referral? Who will chase this referral up? Does the client need to attend regular checkups? Would the client need support at health appointments? Who will provide this support? What type of reasonable adjustments are necessary on the part of the GP, Nurses, hospital etc to enable the individual to receive the treatment or investigation required?

4. When will these actions be taken? (Time frame)

Indicate timeframe for each of the actions you agreed with the client. This ensure momentum and focus

5. How would you know that these actions have been taken? How do you measure health outcomes? Set review dates to update the HAP. How frequently you review HAP will depend on the dynamics in the client's health needs. HAP should be an agenda item at any Person Centred Planning meeting. This way, the client's health needs are discussed in relation to other important issues in the client's life.

There is an argument that primary care professionals, especially GP should take the lead in developing HAP for People with learning disabilities. This writer takes the view that people who know an individual well e.g. Key workers, parents/family, LD professionals (Health Facilitators) are better placed to support the individual to clearly identify and articulate his/her health needs. As already stated in this dissertation Health Facilitators especially unpaid carers and untrained Support Workers would need appropriate trainings to enable them discharge this role effectively. For instance, Health Facilitators need to be aware of what health services/professionals are relevant to health issues that affect their cared for person.

Below is a sample and guide.

Common heath issues and relevant health care professionals

Health Issue	Relevant health Professionals
Medication	GP British National Formulary BNF Psychiatrist (If involved)
Eye & Vision, Hearing	GP Practice Nurse Optician Speech & Language Therapist Audiology clinic

Oral and dental	Dentist Oral Hygienist
Breathing difficulties	GP NHS Direct 999
Epilepsy	GP Neurologist Epilepsy Specialist Nurse
Chest infection	GP Speech and Language Therapist
Diabetes	GP Diabetes Specialist Nurse Practice Nurse District Nurse (if insulin dependent and unable to administer and monitor effect and blood glucose levels)
Foot Health	Chiropodist Podiatrist
High Cholesterol	GP Practice Nurse Dietician
High Blood pressure	GP

	Practice Nurse
Mental health : e.g. Depression Anxiety Psychosis Personality difficulties Obsession	GP LD Psychiatrist Mainstream Psychiatrist Mental health Nurses Psychology
Thyroid problem	GP
Behaviour difficulties	Psychologist Behaviour Therapist Psychiatrist
Anger problem	Psychologist Psychiatrist
Dementia	GP Psychiatrist Psychologist
Malnutrition	GP Dietician
Nails and foot health	Chiropodist, podiatrist, foot health clinic
Skin Conditions	GP
Obesity	GP

	Dietician
	Leisure Centre
	Physiotherapist
Underweight or malnutrition	GP
	Dietician
Dysphasia (Swallowing problem)	Speech and Language Therapist
Constipation	GP
Bowel/bladder activities e.g. incontinence	GP
	District Nursing
	Continence Advisory
	Urologist
Poor/deteriorating mobility/physical disabilities	GP
	Physiotherapist
	Occupational Therapist
Menstrual dysfunction	GP
	Gynecologist
Sexual Health	GP
	Sexual Health clinic
Pregnancy	GP, Practice Nurse
	Antenatal and Post-natal clinics, Health Visitor, Community Midwife

	Psychologist
Women's health & health screening	GP Sexual Health Advisor/Nurse Practice Nurse
Flu/cold symptoms	GP
Accidents	A&E GP
Health screening	GP Practice Nurse
Health checks	GP Practice Nurse
Deficit in activities of daily living skills & opportunities	Occupational Therapist
Emotional problems e.g loss, separation abuse	GP Psychologist Counseling
Self injurious Behaviour/Self harm	GP Psychiatrist, Psychologist

Please note that this is not by any means an exhaustive list.

Community Learning Disabilities Teams
Community Learning Disabilities Team can provide valuable specialised advice and or inputs in all health needs of people with learning disabilities

especially where individual's social circumstance put them at higher risks of experiencing health inequalities and unmet health needs. Community Learning Disability Nurses can offer valuable inputs in all areas listed above. Health professionals commonly found within CLDTs are:

CLD Nurses	Psychologists
Mental Health Nurses	Behaviour Therapists
Health Care Assistants	Specialist Counselor
Psychiatrists	Speech and Language
Dieticians	Therapists Psychiatrists
Physiotherapists	Art Therapist
Occupational Therapists	Social Workers

However, configuration of these teams varied greatly. Not all of them have the listed professionals.

Training Opportunities often offered by the CLDT

Below are some training which are usually offered to carers and others:

Learning Disabilities Awareness

Challenging Behaviour

Mental Health and Learning Disabilities

Autism Awareness

Epilepsy Awareness/Epilepsy Management

Anger Management

Communication skills for staff and carers

Makaton

Dysphagia

Medication Management

Social Skills training for people with learning disabilities

Healthy Living for people with learning disabilities

Health Facilitation and Health Action Planning

Qualities of a Health Facilitator

From various trainings the writer delivered to people with learning disabilities
and carers on Health Facilitation, the following were identified as essential:

Empathy

Ability to communicate
with relevant people

Good local knowledge or
ability to develop this

Ability to listen

Ability to be assertive

Enthusiasm

Non-judgemental

Someone who does not
takeover

Ability to challenge
barriers and others

Ability to know own
limitation

Ability to demonstrate
respect

I.T skills is useful

Ability to listen

Sense of humour helps

Who can be a Health Facilitator?

Valuing People says it is anybody. However, the following have traditionally
supported people with learning disabilities in this regards

Parents
Siblings/Family member
Spouse
Boyfriend/Girlfriend

Friends
Key workers
LD health professionals
Social Workers

Mental Capacity and Consent to Treatment

What this work has not looked at is the issue of consent to treatment and
Mental Capacity Act 2005. It should be pointed out that though the nature of
individual learning disabilities including communication difficulties, cognitive
impairment, sensory and physical disabilities may make it difficult for
individual to comprehend medical information about their condition and to
take a decision whether or not to accept or refuse a treatment or investigation
on offer. The challenge is on the heath professional to ensure that the

proposed clinical procedure is explained to the individual in ways and format which the individual can understand. In doing this, the health professional may consult with the patient's carers where involved. However, the Act states that no adult can consent for another adult. Mental Capacity Act 2005 makes it unlawful to withhold or neglect a person who lacks capacity to make such decision. The Act stipulates that capacity should be assumed until proven otherwise. Where an individual as been assessed as lacking capacity to consent to a medical treatment or procedure, a best interest decision must be taken by the health professional that is carrying out the procedure. Independent Mental Capacity Advocates IMCA are available locally where an individual who lacks capacity to consent has no next of keen or family involvement. In such cases, IMCA can represent the interest of that individual and work with the health professional that is carrying out the procedure and significant others to reach a *best interest* decision.

Learning Disabilities Nurses have played significant roles in supporting individuals to understand treatment options or specific procedures by investing time and energy in one to one work with the individual using accessible information materials. Learning Disability Nurses are also experienced in supporting other health professionals in making their services accessible to individual with learning disabilities. Speech and Language Therapist can also offer support to health professionals in making information accessible to individuals. Below is an example of Learning Disabilities Nursing intervention:

This is the way we do it.

Jonathan (not real name) is a 71 year old gentleman with mild to moderate learning disabilities. Jonathan lived in a 24 hr staffed residential "home for life" from age of 17 until he was 57 when, under Supported Living, he moved to his own flat where he lived alone with local authority funded care package of 3hrs support daily excluding weekend when he receives no support. The support he receives is for a Support Worker to prompt him around his personal hygiene, work with him to tidy up his flat and help him with his weekly shopping. The support worker also supports him with routine health appointments such as GP and repeat prescriptions. Jonathan has high cholesterol, anxiety, he is frail and he walks with an unstable gait, otherwise Jonathan is healthy and fairly independent in all areas of his daily living.

Jonathan has severe speech impediments. His verbal communication can be very difficult to understand for people who are not familiar with him. Jonathan's behaviour can be challenging at times as he can be verbally and physically aggressive when he feels frustrated by events around him or when a demand is placed on him which he disagrees with.

Jonathan does not like people fussing over him. He is a private man who takes great pride in his environment. He spends time travelling independently on local buses to visit local markets and he is well known and liked in the area.

Jonathan does not like hospitals and is anxious around health professionals and is always resistant to attend any outpatient appointments. He however has very good relationship with his GP who has known Jonathan for many years. Jonathan also has good relationship with his older brother who visits him with his sister-in-law weekly. He also has good relationship with his Key worker who has been working with Jonathan for more than 10 years. In the event of any hospital appointments Jonathan's brother and his Key worker always support him. He had been physically aggressive towards hospital staff when he was admitted to the hospital following a fall some years ago.

Jonathan is independent in most areas of his daily living skills especially his personal hygiene. Jonathan's Key Worker noticed that his left side groin area was swollen and bulging. This was visible when looking at upper part of his trousers. When asked, Jonathan denied there was any problem in the area and he refused to talk about it or to allow a male support worker to see the area. He also refused any suggestion of him going to see his GP for examination.

The Key Worker and his care team were very concerned when over time Jonathan's groin area appeared to be getting bigger. Jonathan continued to hide the problem from his care staff. Attention of his brother was called to this problem and Jonathan still refused to let his brother take a look at his groin area, he also refused to talk to anybody about it. His brother and the carers became more concerned. The brother intensified his visits to Jonathan and managed to persuade him to see the GP with his support. At the GP Jonathan became very resistant to examination, he became agitated and aggressive towards the GP. He was screaming and biting his own hands. With the brother's persistence and support, the GP however managed to have a "few seconds fleeting glance". Though the GP was not able to properly examine Jonathan, suspected *Inguinal Hernia* was diagnosed and Jonathan was referred for specialist investigation and appropriate treatment.

Jonathan's brother and Key Worker supported him to local hospital for the OPD appointment. Again, Jonathan became very agitated and uncooperative during the appointment. The Consultant again could not examine Jonathan and terminated the appointment. Even without any mental capacity assessment, the Consultant concluded that Jonathan had capacity to refuse examination and that his non cooperation was interpreted as refusal. The case was closed and the GP informed.

Jonathan's brother and the Key Worker felt frustrated and helpless in their bid to support Jonathan to receive appropriate investigation and treatment. The brother then decided to write a strongly worded letter to the local Community Learning Disabilities Team. Addressing the letter to the Head of Service, Jonathan's brother expressed his concern and he stressed that in his opinion the NHS was failing his brother and that someone should "do something" to either persuade or force Jonathan to receive treatment. By this time Jonathan's groin area had grown bigger and nobody had been able to have any good look at it except what they could see when he was fully dressed.

The Head of Learning Disabilities Team promptly forwarded Jonathan's case to the Community Learning Disabilities Nursing team as an urgent referral. Jonathan was allocated a male Community LD Nurse (CLDN) who promptly initiated contact with Jonathan's brother and his Key Worker to gather more information.

The CLDN met with Jonathan and his Key Worker who introduced the CLDN to Jonathan. Though, it was decided not to talk about Jonathan's suspected hernia during the first few visits. The rationale was to gently introduce the issue when the CLDN and Jonathan may have formed some therapeutic relationship. The CLDN was introduced to Jonathan as someone who would help him with his health generally.

Jonathan likes doing gentle keep fit exercise in his flat, initial discussion was around this since it was a subject which Jonathan was interested in. Jonathan was also interested in cars, this was also a subject used to break the ice with him. Yet Jonathan became very agitated and aggressive towards the CLDN during the first two visits. The Support Worker was able to support both Jonathan and the CLDN on both occasions without any incident.

After few home visits, the CLDN decided the time was right to ask Jonathan about his bulging groin. When asked, Jonathan again became agitated and made it clear he did not want to talk about the issue. The CLDN did not push Jonathan on this, reassured Jonathan and moved to subject of interest to Jonathan.

In the interim, the CLDN had researched into inguinal hernia among men and had accessed different images of hernia which were readily available on *Google image*. Some images showed hernia patients being examined by doctors in different relaxed positions. The CLDN laminated these images to use as resource when discussing with Jonathan.

During one of the home visits, the CLDN gave the images to Jonathan and encouraged him to look at them. Though, Jonathan refused to take the pictures, the CLDN left them in Jonathan's flat for him to look at his own time. The CLDN decided to give Jonathan space and time to look at the pictures and did not visit or contact him for two weeks.

After about two weeks, Jonathan, having looked at the pictures, requested the CLDN to come and visit him at home. As a matter of priority, the CLDN carried out the home visit. Jonathan Key Worker was present during the visit. Jonathan invited the CLDN to his room and showed his groin to the CLDN. The hernia was strikingly similar to those in laminated images which the CLDN had given to Jonathan. The protrusion in Jonathan's groin was big and grouse. Jonathan was clearly worried about it and he quickly asked the CLDN if it was cancer. Apparently, Jonathan's best female friend had died at local hospital of cervical cancer just few years before and Jonathan used to visit her at the hospital before her death. Jonathan had then learnt to associate hospitals with death. Despite CLDN approaching the issues very sensitively, Jonathan still became distressed and constantly saying to himself "I don't want to die, I don't want to die, I've cancer". CLDN and Jonathan spent the next two months talking about Jonathan's hernia, using different images of hernia patients which were freely available on the internet.

The focus was on managing Jonathan's anxieties around his hernia and reassuring him that with treatment he would be alright. The CLDN was visiting Jonathan at least weekly, but often twice weekly to keep the momentum. Jonathan and the CLDN developed good trusting therapeutic relationship and Jonathan started to look forward to the home visits. However, Jonathan was persistent that he did not want an 'operation' or hospital admission. Though, he was clear that he would like the doctor to "make the hernia go away". Jonathan admitted that the hernia was limiting his mobility and preventing him from enjoying his usual activities.

Jonathan agreed to another Outpatient appointment at the local hospital. The CLDN quickly liaised with the GP and the Consultant and informed them of Jonathan's decision.

Jonathan saw the same Consultant he saw before. The Consultant was surprised at Jonathan's level of cooperation and sense of humour. The Consultant confirmed diagnosis of hernia and advised Jonathan that he would need an operation to repair it. At the mention of the word "operation" Jonathan again became agitated, he started screaming and he needed reassurance to settle. Jonathan was supported to the appointment by the CLDN, Jonathan's brother and the Support Worker.

It quickly became apparent to the CLDN that Jonathan was very scared about his condition. He was even more petrified of having a surgical operation. Though, he wanted the hernia which he called 'hernie' to "go away". Despite intensive contact and inputs from the CLDN Jonathan remained very anxious and resistant to any full examination of his hernia. He also at a stage refused to go for hospital appointments

The CLDN quickly arranged a Strategy Meeting which was attended by Jonathan's brother and his key worker. Also invited were a Clinical Psychologist, Psychiatrist and Social Worker. At the meeting the CLDN presented an update on his contacts with Jonathan and his nursing assessment so far. The Clinical Psychologist advised that since Jonathan wanted the hernia to "go away", but rather petrified of the word 'Operation', we should look at alternative words which are less frightening to use when discussing the issues with him. The meeting agreed on "repair", "make it better", "cut it and tuck it back in", "sort it out". Example of sentences could be "the doctor will repair your hernie", "your nurse is coming to see you on Friday to talk about how the doctor can make your hernie better" etc. The focus would also be on the CLDN offering Jonathan the opportunities to talk about his anxieties around his hernia and the proposed repair. An intervention plan based on these points was put together at the meeting. All staff who work with Jonathan including his brother were advised to adopt the new language in all their discussions or contact with him to ensure consistency. This strategy had a significant impact on Jonathan's attitude as he became more receptive and willing to discuss his 'hernie' more openly and he was more cooperative with his CLDN,

The CLDN liaised closely with the Consultant Surgeon and the hospital and physically supported Jonathan to attend all pre-operation assessments appointments. As Jonathan had an intense fear of hospital generally, every appointment needed careful planning to ensure Jonathan's anxiety was managed and for his appointment to go smoothly. The CLDN also needed to do desensitisation work with Jonathan by supporting him to visit the hospital coffee shops, do walk about and familiarise self with the hospital environment. Every pre operation appointment which Jonathan successfully attended was an achievement for him personally and a motivation to attend the next.

Making a case for reasonable adjustment, the CLDN put a case for Jonathan to be fast tracked on the hernia repair waiting list to minimise the suspense and the associated anxiety that could undo all the work that had been put in place so far. The waiting list at the time was 10 months. The hospital fast tracked Jonathan and reduced the wait to five months.

On the day of the surgery, Jonathan requested his CLDN to accompany him him up to the theatre. The Surgeon, Anesthetist and the Nursing team were great with Jonathan. The Surgeon and Anesthetist spend good time with Jonathan explaining the procedure and what would happen during and after the operation to Jonathan while avoiding the word "operation" which both had been informed Jonathan found frightening. Jonathan coped very well throughout his meeting with both. Consulting with Jonathan's brother, Key Worker and the CLDN, the Surgeon concluded that it was in Jonathan's best interest for his hernia to be repaired. Jonathan was found not to have capacity to consent. A best interest form was completed by the surgeon.

At a point when Jonathan was waiting to be wheeled to the theater, He became very anxious and refused to cooperate with the nursing team when they wanted to take his vital observations. At Jonathan's request, the observations were carried out by the CLDN with the permission of the hospital nursing team. Jonathan quickly regained his sense of humour and he entertained the team all the way as he was wheeled to the theatre.

Jonathan successfully had his hernia repair. Jonathan was very happy with the outcome. His brother commented that he was amazed at how the CLDN had worked with his brother and that what the CLDN had done was a "miracle". The brother also commented that in his experience, this was the first time someone actually listened to Jonathan.

Jonathan was discharged from the hospital the following day and he returned back to his full functional ability within two weeks. Jonathan was delighted that his 'hernie' had disappeared. The CLDN liaised with the District Nursing team, the GP and Jonathan's Key worker post discharge to ensure that

Jonathan's wound was dressed regularly and pain killers and other medications were taking as prescribed. The CLDN also arrange for OT bathroom assessment and advice for Jonathan during this period. The CLDN liaised with the Social Worker to ensure that Jonathan's Care Package was increased to provide extra support hours while he recovered.

Comments:

It is important to point out that Jonathan's case is not in any way unique. It is typical of how Learning Disabilities Nurses work creatively to ensure that the health needs of people with learning disabilities are met. CLDNs case load often comprise of clients with various health issues – diabetes, obesity, epilepsy, thyroid problem, hormonal problem, women's health problems, sensory problems, various mental health problems etc to mention a few. These clients live in different social situation from those who completely live on their own with minimum or no care package, to those who live in supported living sheltered accommodation as well as those who live with carers, often single elderly parents. CLDN provide invaluable inputs in all these cases and situations.

National developments:

Since 2006 when this work was first completed, the issue of health inequalities which people with learning disabilities experience has attracted some national attention and the following documents have been released:

- *Equal Treatment: closing the gap*: a Report by the Disability Right Commission on the formal inquiry into physical health inequalities experience of people with mental health problems and or learning disabilities (2006).

- *Death by indifference* (March 2007): A Mencap publication which describes the experience of six people with learning disabilities who died whilst under the care of the NHS. The Report highlighted institutional discrimination within the NHS, and people with a learning disability getting poor healthcare.

- *Healthcare for all* (2008): Report of Independence Inquiry into Access to healthcare for people with learning disabilities. Sir Jonathan Michael

- *Valuing People Now: a new three year Strategy for people with learning disabilities* (DH December 2007)

References

- Acheson D (2000) Round Table Discussion: Health inequalities impact assessment. In <u>Bulletin of the World Health Organisation</u> vol. 78 no. 1

- Alborz A, McNally R, Swallow A & Glendinning C (2004) <u>From the Cradle to the Grave: A literature review of access to health care for people with learning disabilities across the lifespan</u> NHS Service Delivery and Organisation R & D (NCCSDO)

- Alborz A (2005) <u>The role of health check programmes in improving access to mainstream NHS healthcare services for people with learning disabilities</u> National Primary Care Research and Development Centre

- Atherton H (2005) A brief history of learning disability. In <u>NHS QIS GIRT V1.0</u>

- Barr O, Gilgunn J, Kane T & Moore G (1999) Health Screening for people with learning disabilities by a community learning disabilities by a community learning disability nursing service. In Northern Ireland in Journal of Advanced Nursing 29: pp.1482-91

- Barnes C (1999) Exploring Disability: A Sociological introduction Cambridge: Polity Press

- Bond L, Kerr M, Dunstan F & Thapar A (1997) Attitude of general practitioners towards healthcare for people with intellectual disability and factors underlying these attitudes. In Journal of Intellectual Disability Research Vol. 41 No. 5 pp.391-400

- Burns R (2000) Introduction to research methods London: Sage

- Bowling A (2002) Research Methods in Health: investigating health and health services Buckingham: Open University Press

- Bouras, N. & Holt, G. (2000) Planning and provision of psychiatric services for people with mental retardation. In The New Oxford Textbook of Psychiatry, vol. 2 (eds M. G. Gelder, J. J. Lopez-Ibor & N. C. Andreasen), pp. 2007–2012. Oxford: Oxford University Press.

- Caan W, Luchmiah J Thompson K & Toocaram J (2005) Health facilitation in primary care. In Primary Health Care Research and Development Vol. 6 pp 348-355 Edward Arnold Publishers

- Clarke A (1999) Evaluation Research: An Introduction to Principles, methods, and Practice London Sage

- Cocks E (2002) Evaluation of quality in learning disability services in D Race (ed.) Learning Disability: A Social Approach London: Routledge

- Cole A (2006) People with learning disabilities from minority ethnic communities in Newham: Survey Report (Unpublished report for Newham Partnership Board)

- Department of Health (1995) <u>Health of the nation: A strategy for people with learning disabilities</u> London: Crown Press
- Department of Health (1998) <u>Signposts for Success in Commissioning and Providing Health Services for People with Learning Disabilities</u> London: Crown Press
- Department of Health (1999) <u>Once a Day: one or more people with learning disability are likely to be in contact with your Primary Healthcare Team, how can you help them?</u> London: Crown Press
- Department of Health (2001) Valuing People: <u>A New Strategy for Learning Disability for the 21st Century</u> London: Crown Press
- Department of Health (2002) <u>Action for Health – Health Action Plans and Health Facilitation, Detailed Good Practice Guidance on Implementation for Learning Disability Partnership Boards</u> London: Crown Press
- Department of Health (2004) <u>Choosing Health? A consultation on action to improve people's health</u> London: Department of Health
- Disability Right Commission (2006) <u>Equal Treatment: Closing the Gap, Interim Report of a Formal Investigation into Health inequalities,</u> Disability Right Commission
- Earwaker S & Todd M (1995) Service for people with learning disability. In M Todd & T Gilbert (eds) <u>Learning Disabilities: Practice Issues in Health Settings</u> London: Routledge.
- Emerson E (2005) Models of service delivery. In G Grant et al (eds.) <u>Learning Disability: A Life Cycle Approach to Valuing People</u> Maidenhead: Open University Press

- Fink A (1998) <u>Conducting research Literature Reviews: From Paper to the Internet</u> London Sage Publications

- Flynn (2002) Commentary on M Lindsey (2002) article: Comprehensive health care services for people with learning disabilities. In <u>Advances in Psychiatry</u> (2002) Vol. 8 p. 147-148

- Fyson R (2005) Commissioning and Strategic Change in the context of a White Paper on Learning Disabilities. In <u>Research Finding register Summary</u> No. 1394 23 March <u>www.refer.nhs.uk/viewrecord.asp?ID=1394&print=1</u>

- Gardner J & Chapman M (1993) <u>Developing staff competencies for supporting People with Developmental Disabilities: Orientation Book</u>, Baltimore Paul Brookes Publishing

- Gilbert P (2003) Social care services and the social perspective. In <u>Psychiatry</u> Vol. 2 No. 9 September Medicine Publishing Company

- Gilbert J & Rose S (1998) Commissioning and Providing Services. In T Thompson & P Mathias (eds.) <u>Standards and Learning Disability</u> Second London: Edition Bailliere Tindall

- Gilbert P (2006) Social Care services and the Social Care Perspective. In <u>St Georges University of London Learning About intellectual Disabilities and Health on line</u> http:/www.intellectualdisabilty.info/values/social_care_pg.html

- Graham H (2004) <u>Socialeconomic Inequalities in the UK: Evidence of Patterns and Determinants, a short report for the Disability Rights Commission</u>, Lancaster: University Institute for Health Research

- Graham H & Kelly M (2004) Health inequalities: concepts frameworks and policy. In <u>NHS Health Development Agency Briefing paper</u>, Health development Agency <u>www.hda.nhs.uk</u>

- Gravestock, S. & Bouras, N. (1997) Survey of services for adults with learning disabilities. <u>*PsychiatricBulletin*</u>, 21, 197–199.

- Gray D (2004) <u>Doing research in the real world</u> London: Sage

- Gate B (1997) Understanding learning disability. In B Gate (ed.) <u>Learning Disability</u> Third edition New York: Churchill Livingstone

- Greig R (2003) The New Government Policy in England: A Change of Direction. In <u>Psychiatry</u> Vol. 2 No. 8 August, Medicine Publishing Company

- Greig R (2005) <u>The Story so far…*Valuing People:* A New Strategy for Learning Disability for the 21st Century, Long Report</u>, Valuing People Support Team

- Hatton C, Emerson E & Lobb C (2004) <u>Evaluating the Impact of Valuing People Report of Phase 1: A Review of Existing National Dataset</u> Lancaster: University Institute for Health research

- Hart C (1998) <u>Doing a Literature Review</u> London: Sage

- Hart S (1998) Learning-disabled people's experience of general hospitals. In <u>British Journal of Nursing</u> Vol. 7 No. 8

- Healthcare Commission (2005) <u>Draft three-year strategic plan for assessing and encouraging improvement in the health and healthcare of adults with learning disabilities 2006-2009</u>, November, Commission for healthcare audit and Inspection

- Heller R & Hindle T (1998) <u>Essential Manager's Manual</u> London: Dorling Kindersley

- Hollins S et al (1998) Mortality in People with learning disability: risks, causes and death certification findings in London. In Developmental Medicine & Child Neurology Vol.40 p50-56

- Hortwitz S M, Kerker B D, Owen P L & Zigler E (2000) The Health Status and Needs of people with mental retardation, Newhaven: Yale University School of Medicine and Special Olympics. www.specialolympics.org

- Howatson J (2005) Health action for people with learning disabilities. In Nursing Standard vol.19, no. 43 p.51-57

- Juke M (2002) Health facilitation in learning disability: a new specialist role. In British Journal of Nursing May 23-June 12 Vol. 11 No. 10; and ProQuest Nursing & Allied Health Sources p. 694

- Juke M & Bollard M (2002) Health Facilitator in Learning Disability are important roles. In British Journal of Nursing March 14-March 27 Vol. 11 No. 5; and ProQuest Nursing & Allied Health Sources p. 297

- Kawachi I, Subramanian S V & Almeida-Filho N (2002) A glossary for health inequalities Journal of Epidemiology and Community Health 56, pp 647-652, downloaded from http://jech.bmjjournals.com/cgi/content/full/56/9/647 on 16/4/06

- Kelly A (2000) Working with Adult a with a Learning Disability Bicester: Speechmark Publishing Ltd

- Kerr M (2004) Improving the general health of people with learning disabilities. In Advances in Psychiatric Treatment Vol. 10 p. 200-2006

- Keywood K & Flynn (2003) Healthcare Decision-Making by adults with intellectual disabilities: some lever to changing practice. In Psychiatry Vol 2 No. 8 August The Medicine Publishing Company

- Learning Disability Health Task Group (2003) My Health Matters: Health Action Plan framework Newham Partnership for People with Learning Disabilities (Unpublished document)

- Lin J, Yen C & Wu J (2005) Importance and satisfaction of preventive health strategies in institutions for people with intellectual disabilities: a perspective of institutional directors. In Research in Developmental Disabilities vol. 26 pp. 267-280 accessed on line http://www.sciencedirect.com

- Lawton A (1999) Strategic Management in A Rose & A Lawton (eds.) Public Services Management Harlow: Financial Times Prentice Hall

- Lindsey M (2002) Comprehensive health Care services for people with learning disabilities. In Advances in Psychiatric Treatments vol. 8, pp. 138-148

- Mackean S et al (1999) Primary Health Care for Adults with Learning Difficulties Publisher unknown

- Martin G, Philip L, Bates L & Warwick J (2004) Evaluation of a nurse led annual review of patients with severe intellectual disabilities, needs identified and needs met, in a large group practice. In Journal of Learning Disabilities London: Sage

- Mencap (1998) The NHS – Health for all? People with learning disabilities and Health Care UK Mencap

- McCray J & Carter S (2002) A study to determine the qualities of a learning disabilities practitioner. In British Journal of Nursing Vol. 11 pp. 1380-1388

- McCray J (2004) Interprofessional practice and learning disability nursing. In ProQuest Nursing & Allied Health Source pp. 1335

- McGill P (2005) Models of Community Care in the UK: Past and Present. In <u>Learning Disability Review</u> vol. 10 no. 1 Brighton: Pavilion Publishing Ltd.

- Mckenzie F (2005) The roots of Biomedical diagnosis. In G Grant, P Goward, M Richardson & P Ramcharan (eds.) <u>Learning Disability: A Life Cycle Approach to Valuing People</u> Maidenhead: Open University Press

- Mullin L (2005) <u>Management and Organisational Behaviour</u> Seventh Edition London: FT Prentice Hall

- Murray C J L, Gakidou E E, & Frenk J (1999) Health inequalities and social group differences: what should we measure? In <u>Bulletin of the World Health Organisation</u> vol. 77, no. 7 WHO

- NHS Service Delivery and Organisation (SDO) (2004) Access to Healthcare for people with Learning Disabilities. In <u>Access to Healthcare Briefing Paper</u> July NHS SDO R&D

- Nocon A & Qureshi H (1996) <u>Outcomes of Community Care for Users and Carers</u> Buckingham: Open University Press

- Northway R (2001) Poverty as a practice issue for learning disability in <u>British Journal of Nursing</u> London: October, vol. 10, no. 18 pp. 1186

- Parrish A & Styring L (2003) Nurses' role in the developments in learning disability care. In British Journal of Nursing Vol. 8 No.12(17) pp.1043-7.

- Perini A (2000) Development of Health Service Policy for people with learning disability. In the United Kingdom in Hong Kong Journal of Psychiatry Vol.10 No.4 pp. 18-21

- Peters J & Goyder L (2006) Health inequalities in Public Health. The University of Sheffield http://www.shef.ac.uk/scharr/esctions/ph/research/h_i article accessed on 16/04/2006

- Pratt H Pratt H, Nicholls C Scior K & Baum (2005) Evaluation of the Newham Health Action Planning Pilot Newham Community Health Team for People with Learning Disability

- Quthwaite S (2003) The importance of leardership in the development of an integrated team. In Journal of Nursing Management, Vol 11, pp 371-376

- Race D (2002) The historical context. In Race D (ed.) Learning Disability: A Social Approach London: Routledge

- Russell L (2006) Developing health resources with the help of people with Downs syndrome. In Learning Disability Practice May Vol. 9 No.4, pp. 16-18 London: RCN

- Sanderson H (2003) Person centred planning. In G Gates (ed.) Learning Disabilities: Towards Inclusion, fourth edition, Churchill Linvingstone

- Saunders M (2001) Concept of health and disability. In J Thompson & S Pickering (eds.) <u>Meeting the Health Needs of People who have a Learning Disability</u> Edinburgh: Bailliere Tindall

- Shaughnessy P & Cruse S (2001) Health promotion with people who have learning disability. In J Thompson & S Pickering (eds.) <u>Meeting the Health Needs of People who have a Learning Disability</u> Edinburgh: Bailliere Tindall

- Styring L & Grant G (2005) Maintaining a commitment to quality. In G Grant, P Goward, M Richardson, P Ramcharan (eds.) <u>Learning Disabilities: A Life Cycle Approach to Valuing People</u> Maidenhead: Open University Press

- Townsend P & Davidson N (1982) (eds.) <u>Inequality in Health: The Black Report</u> London: Penguin Books Ltd

- Turk V & Burchell S (2003) Developing and Evaluating Personal Health Records for Adults with Learning Disabilities. In Tizard Learning Disability Review vol.8 no. 4 October Brighton: Pavilion Publishing Ltd

- Turner S (2001) Health Needs of people who have learning disability. In J Thompson & S Pickering (eds.) <u>Meeting the Health Needs of People who have a Learning Disability</u> Edinburgh: Bailliere Tindall

- Styring L & Grant G (2005) Maintaining a Commitment to Quality. In G Grant, P Goward, M Richardson, P Ramcharan (eds.) <u>Learning Disability: A Life Cycle Approach to Valuing People</u> Maidenhead: Open University Press

- US Department of health and Human Services (2002) <u>Closing the Gap: a National Blueprint to Improve the Health of Persons with</u>

Mental retardation, Report of the Surgeon General's Conference on Health Disparities and Mental Retardation US Public Health Service

- Whitehead S (1992) The social origin of normalisation. In H Brown & H Smith (eds.) Normalisation: A Reader for the Nineties London: Routledge

- Whitehead M (2000) The concepts and principles of equity and health Copenhagen: World Health Organisation Regional Office for Europe

- Williamson A (2004) Improving services for people with learning disabilities.In Nursing Standard vol. 18, no. 24 pp. 43-51 January

- Wolfenberg W (1972) The Principle of normalisation in human management services. Toronto: National institute of mental retardation

- Woodward A & Kawachi I (2000) Why reduce health inequalities? in Journal of Epidemiology. Community Health Jech online vol. 54 no. 12 pp. 923
  http://jech.bmjjournals.com/cgi/content/full/54/12/923

- Young A & Chesson R (2005) Stakeholders' views on measuring outcomes for people with learning disabilities. In Health and Social Care in the Community vol. 14 no. 1 pp.17-25 Blackwell Publishing Ltd

Notes

Notes

Notes

CPSIA information can be obtained at www.ICGtesting.com
Printed in the USA
BVOW03s2221151013

333865BV00013B/577/P